Issues in Supportive Care of Cancer Patients

Cancer Treatment and Research

WILLIAM L McGUIRE, *series editor*

Livingston RB (ed): Lung Cancer 1. 1981. ISBN 90-247-2394-9.

Bennett Humphrey G, Dehner LP, Grindey GB, Acton RT (eds): Pediatric Oncology 1. 1981. ISBN 90-247-2408-2.

DeCosse JJ, Sherlock P (eds): Gastrointestinal Cancer 1. 1981. ISBN 90-247-2461-9.

Bennett JM (ed): Lymphomas 1, including Hodgkin's Disease. 1981. ISBN 90-247-2479-1.

Bloomfield CD (ed): Adult Leukemias 1. 1982. ISBN 90-247-2478-3.

Paulson DF (ed): Genitourinary Cancer 1. 1982. ISBN 90-247-2480-5.

Muggia FM (ed): Cancer Chemotherapy 1. ISBN 90-247-2713-8.

Bennett Humphrey G, Grindey GB (eds): Pancreatic Tumors in Children. 1982. ISBN 90-247-2702-2.

Costanzi JJ (ed): Malignant Melanoma 1. 1983. ISBN 90-247-2706-5.

Griffiths CT, Fuller AF (eds): Gynecologic Oncology. 1983. ISBN 0-89838-555-5.

Greco AF (ed): Biology and Management of Lung Cancer. 1983. ISBN 0-89838-554-7.

Walker MD (ed): Oncology of the Nervous System. 1983. ISBN 0-89838-567-9.

Higby DJ (ed): Supportive Care in Cancer Therapy. 1983. ISBN 0-89838-569-5.

Herberman RB (ed): Basic and Clinical Tumor Immunology. 1983. ISBN 0-89838-579-2.

Baker LH (ed): Soft Tissue Sarcomas. 1983. ISBN 0-89838-584-9.

Bennett JM (ed): Controversies in the Management of Lymphomas. 1983. ISBN 0-89838-586-5.

Bennett Humphrey G, Grindey GB (eds): Adrenal and Endocrine Tumors in Children. 1983. ISBN 0-89838-590-3.

DeCosse JJ, Sherlock P (eds): Clinical Management of Gastrointestinal Cancer. 1984. ISBN 0-89838-601-2.

Catalona WJ, Ratliff TL (eds): Urologic Oncology. 1984. ISBN 0-89838-628-4.

Santen RJ, Manni A (eds): Diagnosis and Management of Endocrine-related Tumors. 1984. ISBN 0-89838-636-5.

Costanzi JJ (ed): Clinical Management of Malignant Melanoma. 1984. ISBN 0-89838-656-X.

Wolf GT (ed): Head and Neck Oncology. 1984. ISBN 0-89838-657-8.

Alberts DS, Surwit EA (eds): Ovarian Cancer. 1985. ISBN 0-89838-676-4.

Muggia FM (ed): Experimental and Clinical Progress in Cancer Chemotherapy. 1985. ISBN 0-89838-679-9.

Higby DJ (ed): The Cancer Patient and Supportive Care. 1985. ISBN 0-89838-690-X.

Bloomfield CD (ed): Chronic and Acute Leukemias in Adults. 1985. ISBN 0-89838-702-7.

Herberman RB (ed): Cancer Immunology: Innovative Approaches to Therapy. 1986. ISBN 0-89838-757-4.

Hansen HH (ed): Lung Cancer: Basic and Clinical Aspects. 1986. ISBN 0-89838-763-9.

Pinedo HM, Verweij J (eds): Clinical Management of Soft Tissue Sarcomas. 1986. ISBN 0-89838-808-2.

Higby DJ (ed): Issues in Supportive Care of Cancer Patients. 1986. ISBN 0-89838-816-3.

Issues in Supportive Care of Cancer Patients

edited by

DONALD J. HIGBY, M.D.
Chief Hematology/Oncology Service
Baystate Medical Center
Springfield, MA 01199

1986 **MARTINUS NIJHOFF PUBLISHERS**
a member of the KLUWER ACADEMIC PUBLISHERS GROUP
BOSTON / DORDRECHT / LANCASTER

Distributors

for the United States and Canada: Kluwer Academic Publishers, 101 Philip Drive, Assinippi Park, Norwell, MA 02061, USA
for the UK and Ireland: Kluwer Academic Publishers, MTP Press Limited, Falcon House, Queen Square, Lancaster LA1 1RN, UK
for all other countries: Kluwer Academic Publishers Group, Distribution Center, P.O. Box 322, 3300 AH Dordrecht, The Netherlands

Library of Congress Cataloging in Publication Data

```
Issues in supportive care of cancer patients.

   (Cancer treatment and research ; CTAR 30)
   Running title: Issues in supportive care.
   Includes index.
   1. Cancer--Palliative treatment.  2. Cancer--
Patients--Rehabilitation.  3. Cancer--Treatment--
Complications and sequelae.  I. Higby, Donald J.
II. Title: Issues in supportive care.  III. Series:
Cancer treatment and research ; v. 30.  [DNLM:
1. Neoplasms--therapy.  W1 CA693 v.30 / QZ 266 I865]
RC262.I83  1986        616.99'406          86-12421
ISBN 0-89838-816-3
```

ISBN 0-89838-816-3 (this volume)
ISBN 90-247-2426-0 (series)

PRINTED IN THE NETHERLANDS

For my patients, who continue to teach me

Contents

VIII

Series preface

Where do you begin to look for a recent, authoritative article on the diagnosis or management of a particular malignancy? The few general oncology textbooks are generally out of date. Single papers in specialized journals are informative but seldom comprehensive; these are more often preliminary reports on a very limited number of patients. Certain general journals frequently publish good indepth reviews of cancer topics, and published symposium lectures are often the best overviews available. Unfortunately, these reviews and supplements appear sporadically, and the reader can never be sure when a topic of special interest will be covered.

Cancer Treatment and Research is a series of authoritative volumes which aim to meet this need. It is an attempt to establish a critical mass of oncology literature covering virtually all oncology topics, revised frequently to keep the coverage up to date, easily available on a single library shelf or by a single personal subscription.

We have approached the problem in the following fashion. First, by dividing the oncology literature into specific subdivisions such as lung cancer, genitourinary cancer, pediatric oncology, etc. Second, by asking eminent authorities in each of these areas to edit a volume on the specific topic on an annual or biannual basis. Each topic and tumor type is covered in a volume appearing frequently and predictably, discussing current diagnosis, staging, markers, all forms of treatment modalities, basic biology, and more.

In Cancer Treatment and Research, we have an outstanding group of editors, each having made a major commitment to bring to this new series the very best literature in his or her field. Martinus Nijhoff Publishers has made an equally major commitment to the rapid publication of high quality books, and world-wide distribution.

Where can you go to find quickly a recent authoritative article on any major oncology problem? We hope that Cancer Treatment and Research provides an answer.

WILLIAM L. MCGUIRE
Series Editor

Volume preface

'Supportive care' is a protean subject. During the past decade, our society seems to have gone from a position of great optimism regarding the imminent possibility of cure for cancer to a position in which the 'inevitability' of death for the majority of patients with this disease again governs many decisions. Whole cottage industries have sprung up around 'death and dying'; a new profesion, 'thanatology', vies for clients who need help in the transition from life to death. More disturbing, perhaps, is the attitude expressed by many physicians in training when a cancer patient is admitted to a service; the first question asked of the attending is whether the patient should be resuscitated if perchance he or she should undergo a cardiac arrest while in the hospital.

The effects of these attitudes on the lay public is far more apparent in a community teaching hospital than in a 'cancer center' where the more articulate spokespersons for the oncologic disciplines dwell. The people who seek care in such well known institutions are distinguished primarily by the attitude that they are willing to go to great lengths if there is even a slight chance of cure or prolonged remission. Their counterparts who do not seek such care are generally more fatalistic and less sophisticated; but there is a growing minority of misinformed individuals who have concluded that insofar as medicine is scientific, it must perforce be inhuman. It is disheartening to hear from a middle-aged woman with metastatic breast cancer clinically limited to bone, who is in a great deal of pain after responding to, and then relapsing from, hormonal therapy, that she does not wish to take chemotherapy because she is more interested in the quality of life rather than its duration. It is also sad to see the fatalism among one's professional colleagues who discourage their patients with 'incurable' malignancies from entering clinical trials because participation will not cure them, and may cause significant toxicity.

We seem to be going through a period of retrenchment just as we enter a new era of biologic response modifiers, of oncogenes, of the discovery and understanding of mechanisms of drug resistance. Extremely important questions need to be answered in large-scale clinical trials, some of which fail because of lack of patient accrual, while others take entirely too long to complete, sometimes becoming irrelevant before the final analysis. As more and more questions are posed, fewer and fewer patients enter trials.* Wittes recently concluded that current prospects for increasing the number of patients entering clinical trials is not very bright, and therefore it is necessary to reduce the number of trials. To reduce the number of trials, it will be necessary to coordinate the activities of the large groups at the level of the federal government. While all this is going on, the nationwide supply of oncologists is rapidly reaching a saturation point. Oncologists in practice must compete for patients; they must evaluate the return on time invested in different activities. Trials created and coordinated at the level of the federal government and run by the large cooperative groups are getting more and more complex, and larger amounts of unrecompensed time must be invested by the practicing oncologist to enroll patients on these trials. It is no wonder that the number of patients entering trials is decreasing, but it is also unlikely that further centralization will stem this tide.

Classical economic theory states that consumers can be persuaded to buy one of several very similar products if that product is seen as sufficiently differentiated from the rest (even though it may not be). Product differentiation accounts for why some people drive Chevrolets, and others drive Fords. It is time our National Cancer Institute tackles the perceptual problem at the level of the lay public, rather than by attempting to use moral suasion on practicing oncologists. One large tobacco company writes clever essays which appear in national magazines, the subtle message being that smokers have as much right to smoke as non-smokers have not to smoke, and there is something impolite about a non-smoker who wishes to breath smoke-free air. Surely we could convince the public that it would be to everyone's best interest if cancer patients requested clinical trials rather than 'standard therapy'.

Clinical trials improve the likelihood that patients are appropriately treated; they guarantee that the patient will receive a treatment which is very nearly equivalent to the best conventional treatment available for that disease, at that stage in its evolution. Clinical trials assure that there will be central review of data – a free consultation! Clinical trials assure that if someone discovers a miracle cure for a particular disease, the patient enrolled on a trial for that disease will be in the vanguard of those who hear about it first.

---

* Wittes, Robert E., Friedman, Michael A., Simon, Richard. 1986. Some thoughts on the future of clinical trials in cancer. Cancer Treat. Rep. 70(2):241–250.

A person with fatal cancer bears a hatred for the malignant growth which promises his destruction. What better revenge than to contribute to its eventual elimination? My children and grandchildren will have a better chance of 'beating' cancer if I now participate in a clinical trial than if I don't.

Some people argue that participation in clinical trials will raise the total cost of health care to society. Actually, the argument could be more easily defended that the person being treated as part of a clinical trial utilizes society's resources much more efficiently than his counterpart who is treated with 'standard' therapy, off a trial. For relatively little added expenditure, not only is the patient treated, but advances in treatment come about sooner than they would otherwise, saving money in both the short and the long run.

In the current volume, several topics are addressed which have to do with the palliation of the cancer patient. Some of the areas are quite traditional: Klein's chapter on Hospice care; Harbaugh and Saunder's chapter on Neurosurgical options in cancer pain management. Other chapters deal with areas which are quite new, but at present, largely used in palliation: White and Antman's chapter on Regional chemotherapy; Scott's chapter on the use of hyperthermia for treatment of malignant disease.

Our ability to palliate and support the cancer patient has improved dramatically during the last fifteen years. Our improved understanding in biology, psychology, drug action, sociology, and several other fields have allowed us to be increasingly 'scientific' about how we go about relieving pain and suffering in the cancer patient. At the same time, we need to constantly remind ourselves that palliation is necessary because we haven't found the best ways to treat cancer; palliation and supportive care are more worthwhile if in fact these goals are not ends in themselves, but rather, part of an overall strategy to eliminate cancer. Because we can palliate and support better, we have the opportunity to investigate new treatment concepts more adequately.

Its time that professionals and patients alike rekindle the desire to eliminate cancer, using the most effective tool we have, the clinical trial.

I am most appreciative of the efforts of Mrs. Suzanne Bourbonnais in developing this volume.

DONALD J. HIGBY

List of contributors

Karne Antman, M.D., Assistant Professor of Medicine, Dana Farber Cancer Institute, 44 Binney Street, Boston, MA 02115, USA

Jo-Anne M. Bessette, M.D., Hematology/Oncology Service, Baystate Medical Center, 759 Chestnut Street, Springfield, MA 01199, USA

David F. Cella, Ph.D., Instructor in Psychiatry, Department of Psychiatry, Memorial Sloan Kettering Cancer Center, 1275 York Street, New York, NY 10021, USA

Edmond E. Charrette, M.D., Medical Director, New England Rehabilitation Hospital, Rehabilitation Way, Woburn, MA 01801, USA

William M. Davis, M.D., Co-Director, Hematology Laboratory, Chief, Hematology Section, Baystate Medical Center, 759 Chestnut Street, Springfield, MA 01199, USA

Gerald J. Elfenbein, M.D., Associate Professor of Medicine, Medical Director, Bone Marrow Transplant Unit, College of Medicine, University of Florida, Gainesville, FL 32610, USA

Daniel Friedensen, M.D., Director, Psychiatry Consultation Service, Department of Psychiatry, Baystate Medical Center, 759 Chestnut Street, Springfield, MA 01199, USA

Robert E. Harbaugh, M.D., Assistant Professor of Surgery, Section of Neurosurgery, Dartmouth-Hitchcock Medical Center, Hanover, NH 03756, USA

Donald J. Higby, M.D., Chief, Hematology/Oncology Service, Baystate Medical Center, 759 Chestnut Street, Springfield, MA 01199, USA

Sandra Jacoby Klein, M.A., Hospice Specialist, Division of Cancer Control, Jonsson Comprehensive Cancer Center, University of California at Los Angeles, Westwood, CA, USA

John N. Landis, M.D., Chief, Pulmonary Service, Baystate Medical Center, 759 Chestnut Street, Springfield, MA 01199, USA

David M. O'Toole, M.D., Staff Physician, New England Rehabilitation Hospital, Rehabilitation Way, Woburn, MA 01801, USA

H. Ian Robins, M.D., PhD, Assistant Professor of Human Oncology, K4/666 Clinical Science Center, 600 Highland Avenue, Madison, WI 53792, USA

Ellen P. Romsaas, M.S., O.T.R., C.R.C., Program Director for Cancer Rehabilitation, University of Wisconsin Hospital and Clinic, 600 Highland Avenue, Madison, WI 53792, USA

Richard L. Saunders, M.D., Professor of Surgery, Section of Neurosurgery, Dartmouth-Hitchcock Medical Center, Hanover, NH 03756, USA

Ronald S. Scott, M.D., Ph.D., Assistant Professor, Department of Radiation Oncology, University of Washington School of Medicine, 1959 Pacific, Seattel, WA 91436, USA

Richard H. Steingart, M.D., Staff Physician, Hematology/Oncology Service, Baystate Medical Center, 759 Chestnut Street, Springfield, MA 01199, USA

Charles F. White, M.D., Staff Physician, Hematology/Oncology Service, Baystate Medical Center, 759 Chestnut Street, Springfield, MA 01199, USA

1. Hematologic disorders associated with cancer: I. Red blood cell disorders

WILLIAM M. DAVIS

Introduction

Anemia is the most common hematologic abnormality in patients with cancer. Anemia can be defined in several ways including: (1) decrease in red blood cell count, hemoglobin, or hematocrit (concentration measurements); (2) decrease in the red cell volume or Cr^{51} red cell mass. The mechanisms of cancer-related anemia are treated in detail in other reviews (1, 2).

The clinical laboratories today almost invariably utilize multichannel automated instruments for the generation of the 'complete' blood count. The instruments determine the red blood cell count (RBC), the hemoglobin, and the average size of the red cells (MCV*) with precision and accuracy. The instrument reports red cell indices (MCV*, MCH*, MCHC*) as well as a red cell distribution width (RDW) which is the coefficient of variation, expressed as percentage, of the red cell size distribution. This is a measure of anisocytosis. The most useful red cell index is the MCV. On the basis of the MCV, anemias are classified as microcytic, normocytic, or macrocytic. The MCHC is also helpful as a measure of hemoglobinzation of the red blood cells and characterization of a normochromic versus hypochromic state. However, hypochromia, particularly in terms of distribution among individual cells, is best estimated by a careful review of the peripheral blood smear. The hematocrit is electronically computed from the RBC and MCV.

In addition, these instruments determine an accurate white blood count (WBC) and platelet count and report a mean platelet volume (MPV) as a measure of the size distribution of the platelets. The current instruments may supply a three part differential in which the white cells are classified as granulocytes, mononuclear cells, or lymphocytes. In healthy individuals in association with an otherwise normal blood count, this is often sufficient.

---

* MCV = mean cell volume; MCH = mean corpuscular hemoglobin; MCHC = mean corpuscular hemoglobin concentration.

Higby, DJ (ed), Issues in Supportive Care of Cancer Patients. ISBN 0-89838-816-3.
© *1986, Martinus Nijhoff Publishers, Boston. Printed in the Netherlands.*

However, in patients with hematologic disorders, a careful review of the peripheral blood smear including a 100–200 cell differential by a physician or skilled technologist may be essential.

In the careful assessment of a patient with anemia, an estimate of the reticulocyte count (e.g., the corrected reticulocyte index) is a measure of bone marrow function and ability to produce and release red blood cells. On the basis of this index and bone marrow cellularity and morphology, anemias can be classified as hypoproliferative, normoproliferative, or hyperproliferative.

The approach to the patient can be based on either morphology (red cell indices, peripheral blood smear), pathophysiology, or etiologic considerations. In practice, it is usual to evaluate all three with emphasis on the first two. A current or very recent episode of bleeding may lead to an anemia which will be normocytic and normochromic. Such bleeding episodes are most often from the gastrointestinal or genitourinary tract, but can occur in the tracheobronchial tree. Such episodes may be quite apparent and self evident or more obscure unless searched for. In addition to bleeding, bone marrow invasion or hemolysis may be important mechanisms for anemia in patients with underlying cancer. Table 1 lists the major factors which contribute to the anemia in patients with malignant disease.

Hypersplenism is another possible mechanism for anemia in patients with myeloproliferative and lymphoproliferative disorders [3–5]. The major criteria for hypersplenism are: (1) anemia, leukopenia, and thrombocytopenia, or combinations of the above; (2) splenomegaly; (3) adequate or increased marrow production of the blood cell lines depressed peripherally; and (4) response to splenectomy (if performed). The three factors which play a role in hypersplenism appear to be splenic pooling of red blood cells, leucocytes, and platelets, increased plasma volume (pseudoanemia) and shortened red cell survival. If splenectomy is not performed because of medical contraindications, the hypersplenism may respond with improvement after therapy for the underlying hematologic malignancy.

An increased plasma volume has been reported in numerous malignant disorders. It can be seen in patients with splenomegaly, as described earlier,

Table 1. Factors leading to anemia in patients with malignant disease.

Common	Uncommon
Blood loss	Nutritional disturbance
Infection	Impaired renal function
Bone marrow infiltration	Hemolytic anemia
Anemia of chronic disease	Hypersplenism
Hemodilution	Erythrophagocytosis
Marrowimpairment from previous treatment	

and also it has been noted in some patients with monoclonal gammopathies. Finally, an inappropriate increase in antidiuretic hormone is seen as a rare complication of certain tumors, most often small cell carcinoma of the lung. The end result of such increases in plasma volume may be to create a condition of pseudoanemia (normal red cell mass with increased plasma volume) or increase the apparent degree of an associated anemia.

Erythrophagocytosis is a pathological finding seen in the examination of tumors, lymph nodes, or bone marrow, but which is rarely of major specificity or severity except in histiocytic medullary reticulosis (HMR) [6–8]. It seems likely that this is an important cause of the anemia that is seen in this syndrome. In other situations in which erythrophagocytosis has been described, such as T-cell lymphoma, other lymphomas, acute leukemias and multiple myeloma, it is more incidental and not a major factor in the anemia. HMR will be discussed in more detail later in the chapter.

In the following discussion, a variety of different hematologic conditions characterized by anemia will be discussed individually. However, it should be emphasized that multiple causes and factors may be involved in a particular patient. For example, the anemia of chronic disease [9, 10], seen in patients with infection, inflammation, and malignancy, is to a degree present in many patients.

Iron deficiency anemia (IDA) and blood loss

Many patients may bleed chronically and insidiously. The resulting anemia will present as the anemia of iron deficiency. A diagnosis of IDA should be based on a microcytic, hypochromic picture confirmed by red cell indices and peripheral blood smear, low serum ferritin or low serum iron and elevated total iron binding capacity (TIBC) with low saturation (less than 10%), or when suspected but not proven, an assessment of bone marrow iron stores may be helpful. IDA will on occasion be accompanied by a modest elevation of platelet count (greater than $450,000/mm^3$) with microcytic platelets. The most likely source of chronic bleeding is the gastrointestinal tract and a thorough investigation is usually warranted. Chronic blood loss from a gynecological malignancy is not infrequent. Bleeding from renal or bladder tumors also can lead to significant iron deficiency anemia. There are other rarer causes of IDA including iron malabsorption in patients after subtotal or total gastrectomy for carcinoma of the stomach. Obviously, although IDA may respond to iron therapy, the important point is rather the recognition of the tumor and surgical removal or other appropriate treatment. There are circumstances where although a site of chronic blood loss is known, conditions preclude definitive therapy (inoperable cancer, etc.). In these circumstances, iron administration and even blood replacement therapy may be the only logical treatment.

Anemia of chronic disease (ACD)

The anemia associated with chronic disease and inflammation is a frequent finding in patients with underlying malignancy [9, 10]. Characteristically, the anemia is relatively mild with hemoglobin rarely falling below 9.0 g/dl unless other factors are present. The red cell morphology is most frequently normocytic (75% of patients) but sometimes minimally microcytic (25% of patients) may be normochromic or mildly hypochromic. In the latter situation, a distinction between IDA and ACD may be difficult. The iron parameters include a low serum iron and decreased or normal TIBC with subnormal saturation. Serum ferritin should be normal or elevated. The bone marrow aspiration will demonstrate normoblastic erythroid maturation and an increase in reticuloendothelial (RE) iron, unlike the anemia of iron deficiency where iron stores will be absent. In practice, the distinction between this most frequent cause of anemia may be easy or may be uncertain due to conflicting or confusing test results. This form of anemia is generally manifested by a patient with a fairly extensive (often metastatic) tumor rather than a small primary carcinoma. ACD is associated with a slight although demonstrable shortening of red cell survival utilizing CR^{51} labeled patient or normal red cells [11]. Thus, the shortened survival represents an extracorpuscular rather than intracorpuscular defect. The relative sequestration of the iron in the RE system and thus the unavailability of iron for hemoglobin incorporation appears to be the major factor but why this occurs is not entirely clear.

Ferrokinetic studies are of interest [12, 13]. Injection of radiolabeled (Fe^{59}) iron shows prompt and rapid plasma iron clearance and increased and rapid iron incorporation in the circulating red blood cells. However, when the studies are repeated utilizing Fe^{59} labeled hemoglobin there is poor iron incorporation and the iron largely localizes in the RE system (spleen and liver). In summary, the modest shortening of red cell survival compounds the anemia that results from the poor and impaired reutilization of hemoglobin iron. ACD of itself rarely requires therapy and will improve if the underlying malignancy can be treated effectively.

Megablastic anemias

The macrocytic anemias characterized by megaloblastic bone marrow morphologic features are most frequently secondary to either folate or vitamin B12 deficiency [14]. In patients on antifolate or other antimetabolite drugs, a mild anemia with macrocytosis with megaloblastic marrow findings can be seen, e.g. methotrexate, 6-mercaptopurine, 6-thioguanine, cytosine arabinoside, 5-flourouracil.

The increased incidence of gastric carcinoma in patients with Addisonian pernicious anemia is well known, but in a practice rarely seen. Vitamin B12 deficiency infrequently complicates malignant disease. However, in the wake of total gastrectomy for gastric carcinoma or lymphoma, a macrocytic anemia may evolve over time as the patient's vitamin B12 stores are gradually depleted. Unfortunately, few of such patients survive long enough for this to occur. Rarely, lymphomatous disease of the small bowel or occasionally surgical removal of the ileum for tumors may lead to failure of vitamin B12 absorption and to a vitamin B12 deficiency related macrocytic anemia. These will respond to parenteral vitamin B12 therapy.

More frequently, dietary intake of folate may be deficient or inadequate due to poor appetite, nausea, fever or the effects of therapy. Since there are no normal significant stores of folate, a dietary deficiency of folate can occur relatively rapidly. It can be demonstrated in a subclinical state by low serum and/or red cell folate levels. Such a deficiency can also develop due to leukemic or lymphomatous involvement of the small bowel. Patients with head and neck cancer or esophageal carcinoma may have great difficulty eating and thus become overtly folate depleted unless replaced parenterally. Folate deficiency may also predispose to toxicity when antifolate drugs such as methotrexate are used; pharmaceuticals with mild antifolate properties such as trimethoprim-sulfamethoxazole are more likely to cause toxicity when folate deficiency is present. Folic acid deficiency states will respond to folate replacement; theoretically, there may be an enhanced affect on tumor growth, however.

Pure red blood cell aplasia (PRBCA)

This extremely rare form of chronic anemia deserves discussion because of its frequent association with thymomas, both benign and malignant [15–18]. The anemia is normocytic and normochromic with reticulocytopenia. Usually the white blood counts and platelets are normal. Ferrokinetic studies show markedly impaired iron incorporation. No evidence of hemolysis is seen. Bone marrows show normal myeloid elements and megakaryocytes. Decreased and virtually absent erythroid precursors are noted. These are usually basophilic erythroblasts and proerythroblasts rather than more mature cells. An apparent increase in lymphocytes and sometimes plasma cells is seen. The marrow may on occasion be significantly hypocellular with associated moderate neutropenia and thrombocytopenia. An association with hypogammoglobinemia and myasthenia gravis has been reported. An autoimmune hemolytic anemia (AIHA) has also been seen in rare cases. The distinction between malignant or benign thymic tumors is usually clinical and based on its extension and operability rather than on firm morphologic criteria. A patient presenting with PRBCA should have a chest X-ray looking for a thymoma. The CT scan of the chest can be more definitive and will often pick up a thymoma not seen on chest X-ray. A CT scan also is a better measure of the extent and infiltrative characteristics of the tumor.

In patients with PRBCA, a thymic tumor will be found in about 50% of patients, although, in patients with a thymic tumor, PRBCA will be present in about 5%. There are scattered reports of PRBCA in patients with chronic lymphocytic leukemia and other tumors [19, 20]. Whether this is a direct relationship or a fortuitous association is not clear. Strong evidence exists for an autoimmune mechanism in the case of thymoma and PRBCA as extensively reported by Krantz et al. [15, 16]. These studies have shown a serum IgG antibody that reacts with erythroblast nuclei and is cytoxic for erythroblasts in the presence of complement. In some patients a serum factor interferring with the action of erythropoietin has been demonstrated. The reported frequency of other autoimmune disorders such as myasthesia gravis and hypogammoglobulinemia with PRBCA is also most suggestive of an autoimmune basis.

Thymectomy, if possible technically, is the most effective treatment, although in those patients in whom removal is not possible, other therapies such as androgens, corticosteroids, and immunosuppressive agents have provided occasional clinical benefits.

Histiocytic medullary reticulosis (HMR)

This systemic malignancy was first reported in 1939 but has been well documented in numerous subsequent reports [6–8, 21], although it is a relatively rare disorder. The clinical presentation is characterized by fever, anorexia, weight loss, anemia, weakness and a variety of other systemic manifestations. The course is rapidly progressive and usually fatal. There is an extensive invasive proliferation of morphologically atypical histocytes in multiple regions. These include liver, spleen, multiple lymph nodes, and bone marrow. Hepatomegaly, splenomegaly, and lymphadenopathy are frequently seen. The unique and almost invariable characteristic of the disease is intense erythrophagocytosis by histiocytes. The resulting anemia is usually normocytic and normochromic and there is frequently associated leukopenia and thrombocytopenia. Disseminated intravascular coagulation has been reported in a few cases. Although rarely the abnormal histiocytes may be found in the peripheral blood, a tissue diagnosis is usually required. This can be documented by bone marrow aspiration and biopsy. Alternatively, lymph node biopsy will demonstrate the intense histiocytic infiltration and evidence of erythrophagocytosis. The differential diagnosis lies between benign histiocytic proliferation (occasionally virally induced) and malignant disorders such as diffuse large cell lymphoma. Despite early reports, various therapies including steroids have been singularly unsuccessful. Recently more aggressive multiple drug chemotherapeutic therapy appropriate for malignant lymphoma have induced remissions, often transient [22].

Autoimmune hemolytic anemia (AIHA)

In contrast to the modest shortening of red cell survival present in many patients with malignant disease (ACD), a more significant hemolytic process with antibody production and an 'autoimmune' mechanism is clearly evident in certain groups of patients, primarily but not solely those with lymphoproliferative disorders [23, 24]. A major distinction has to be made between those produced by warm active antibodies and those produced by cold active antibodies.

The warm antibody AIHA can be mild and relatively occult or can be a severe life threatening problem. The lymphoproliferative disorders are the most frequent tumors in which this occurs. Diagnosis rests on evidence of hemolysis, a positive Coombs' test with the demonstration of a warm antibody by direct (DAT) and indirect antiglobulin techniques [25], and by evidence of a compensatory marrow response with reticulocytosis and early release of nucleated red blood cells. The peripheral blood smear will demonstrate anisocytosis, poikilocytosis, basophilic stippling and polychromatophilia, and often an occasional nucleated red blood cell (normoblast). Evaluation of the positive antiglobulin reaction (at 37 °C) will demonstrate antibody (IgG usually) with and without complement coating of the red cells in the DAT and often a circulating antibody (indirect test). The antibody has specificity for the rhesus (Rh) system is appropriately tested for, but may occasionally be directed against other red cell antigens [26]. The hemolysis is generally extravascular. Occasionally, when severe and complement induced, there can be evidence of intravascular hemolysis with hemoglobinemia and hemoglobinuria. Survival studies have demonstrated reduction in red cell survival and evidence for splenic sequestration and destruction by the monocytic phagocytes of the RE system (spleen and to some extent liver). In certain patients, such as previously transfused patients, the differential diagnosis would include a subacute or delayed transfusion reaction. Chronic lymphocytic leukemia (CLL) [27] has the highest frequency of AIHA with a significant shortening of survival of patients with this complication. It is estimated that 20–25 % of patients with CLL may show AIHA at some time in their course. Less frequently, AIHA has been seen in patients with lymphoma, Hodgkin's disease and non-Hodgkin's lymphoma, with a reported incidence of 2–3 % in several large series [27–29]. Occasionally, AIHA may preceed the recognition of the underlying leukemia or lymphoma. In the group of patients with AIHA and Hodgkin's disease a significant proportion have been reported showing an anti-I[t] antibody specificity [30]. The best therapy and management program for patient's with AIHA is treatment for the underlying malignancy; when not possible, corticosterpoids, or occasionally even splenectomy, may be useful.

Although AIHA has rarely been reported in most solid tumors, there is a reported association of AIHA with ovarian tumors and often benign dermoid cysts. Studies have failed to demonstrate that the tumor is the source of the antibody, although this is suggested by the recovery from the hemolytic process when the ovarian tumor is removed.

In contrast, cold antibody AIHA is relatively rare and is usually chronic [31, 32]. The anemia, besides its chronicity, is less severe and symptomatically the patients complain of fatigue and malaise. Raynaud's phenomenon is sometimes noted and hemolytic crises can occur. Peripheral blood smears will frequently demonstrate significant red cell agglutination. Tests for cold agglutins will be positive. Positive antiglobulin tests due to coating of the red cells by antibody and complement can be demonstrated. When this test is performed by techniques that do not permit the antibody to disassociate, IgM antibody is most frequently found. Only rarely do IgA and IgG antibodies cause cold agglutinin hemolytic anemia. These patients most frequently demonstrate by serum protein electropheresis a spike in the gamma or beta regions. By immunoelectropheretic techniques, monoclonal antibody can be demonstrated. The cold antibody is most frequently anti-I or anti-i. Cold antibody AIHA is associated with a variety of B-cell disease of the lymphoid system such as non-Hodgkin's lymphoma, chronic lymphocytic leukemia, multiple myeloma, and Waldenstrom's macroglobulinemia.

The clinical severity of the hemolytic process correlates poorly with the titer of cold agglutinins but better with the thermal range of activity of the antibody. As in warm antibody AIHA, treatment of underlying disease is most likely to control the process but the use of corticosteroids and occasionally splenectomy have to be considered.

Microangiopathic hemolytic anemias (MAHA)

This unusual, but striking, form of hemolytic anemia in seen occasionally in patients with cancer, especially metastatic mucin producing carcinomas of the gastrointestinal tract [33–37]. The anemia is frequently severe, symptomatic, and acute. It may present in patients prior to the recognition of a carcinoma. Morphologically, it is characterized by fragmented red cells of several types, with evidence of hemolysis, an active marrow with compensatory erythroid hyperplasia and variable reticulocytosis, and significant thrombocytopenia. The hallmark of the disease is the presence of schistocytes in the peripheral blood smear. These are characteristically 'burr' cells, 'helmet' cells and bizarre red cell fragments. Evidence for hemolysis may include hemoglobinemia, hyperbilirubinemia, decreased haptoglobin, and elevation of the LDH isoenzymes, LDH 1 and LDH 2. The process is clearly extracorpuscular since it affects red cells from the patient as well as from normal donors. Evidence for occult or overt disseminated intravascular coagulation (DIC) can often be found. The exact mechanism of the intravascular fragmentation is not entirely clear. It is suggested that the red cell fragments are produced mechanically as red cells are forced through fibrin strands in areas of microthrombi. Another possible explanation is a direct interaction between localized intravascular tumor cells and the red cells. Finally, a procoagulant action of mucin producing adenocarcinomas may initiate a DIC-like syndrome. MAHA can be seen in patients with widespread metastatic disease, presumably representing multiple tumor emboli and small blood vessel involvement. These tumors in which MAHA is seen include gastric ($\pm 50\%$) bowel tumors, as well as lung [38], breast, prostate and pancreatic carcinomas. This form of anemia is difficult to treat and associated with a high and relatively immediate mortality. Appropriate management includes vigorous blood replacement utilizing packed red blood cells and platelet concentrates. Heparin may occasionally bring about transient benefit. Treatment of the underlying malignancy is the only definite therapy.

There is a similar syndrome in patients under treatment with chemotherapeutic agents, particularly Mitomycin C. This is characterized by MAHA and renal failure [39, 40]. This syndrome often appears later in the course of chemotherapy, when the patient is in a complete or near complete remission. Platelet-aggregating immune complexes have been described in these patients. These do not appear to be antibodies to a Mitomycin-related antigen. The syndrome has been seen primarily in patients with gastric and colon carcinoma. Aggressive supportive therapy is essential in these patients. Reactions to blood transfusions, however, have been reported. Mitomycin C should probably be discontinued although in some patients it has been possible to continue with Mitomycin after the patient had recovered from the syndrome.

Leukoerythroblastic anemia (malignant infiltration of the bone marrow)

This entity, which is seen in patients with infiltration of the marrow by malignant tumors, is by definition a moderate to severe anemia accompanied by the presence of significant numbers of immature red blood cells (reticulocytes, nucleated red cells and occasional early erythroblasts), and a few immature granulocytic cells (usually myelocytes but rarely progranulocytes and myeloblasts) in the peripheral blood [41]. The term 'myelophthisic' anemia is also used but is less descriptive. Usually platelets are moderately to severely reduced in number. The actual level of the white blood count is quite variable. The red cells should reflect moderate to marked anisocytosis and poikilocytosis. Nucleated red cells are almost invariably present. A spectrum of bizarrely shaped red cells is seen. The severity is graded largely in terms of the quantitation of these changes.

These changes can be seen in any malignancy extensively infiltrating the marrow. The degree of these abnormalities varies from patient to patient and does not always correlate with the extent of marrow involvement. 'Crowding out' or marrow replacement may play a major role in leukoery-throblastic anemia, but careful assessment also suggests early release or the lack of control of release of marrow elements into the circulation. The role of extramedullary hematopoeisis is not clear. In some patients the marrow demonstrates significant myelofibrosis with splenomegaly as a reaction to the presence of tumor. The early release of marrow elements may also be related to an 'irritative' reaction of the marrow to the tumor. The same picture can be seen in a number of nonmalignant diseases characterized by marrow replacement such as Gaucher's Disease, idiopathic myelofibrosis, and myelofibrosis secondary to polycythemia vera. The most likely solid tumors to be associated with this particular blood picture are tumors of the breast, prostate, lung, adrenal, thyroid, and kidney with their higher predilection for bone marrow metastasis.

The diagnosis of the leukoerythroblastic anemia is relatively easy and is based first of all on review of the peripheral blood smear and the findings as described above. A bone marrow aspiration may be unsuccessful (dry tap) or may be a sparse specimen which reveals nests of tumor cells. Tumor cells can be distinguished from hematopoetic elements because they tend to be larger (except for megakaryocytes) than the other marrow cells; they vary considerably in size; usually a large central nucleus with hyperchromatic features is seen; and usually one or more prominent nucleoli are noted.

However, when the patient has no established primary tumor, it is often important to know the histology of the tumor cells infiltrating the marrow. An aspirated marrow is not very helpful in this regard, unless the tumor cells are clearly mucus-secreting. For example, it may be quite difficult to distinguish between small cell lung cancer and acute lymphocytic leukemia, or poorly differentiated lymphoblastic lymphoma, on the basis of aspirated marrow. Because of the incidence of 'dry taps' and because of the added information obtained from biopsy, it is prudent to obtain a bone marrow biopsy, rather than an aspirate, when the diagnosis of leukoerythroblastic leukemia is suspected. Bilateral biopsies will further increase the diagnostic yield. The technique for obtaining satisfactory bone marrow needle biopsies is well established and the expected yield and usefulness of the technique is well documented [42].

Patients with leukoerythroblastic anemia usually develop progressive severe pancytopenia consistent with diffuse replacement of bone marrow, and sometimes bone marrow necrosis is seen as a late consequence of marrow involvement by malignant disease.

Leukoerythroblastic syndrome is an ominous sign requiring vigorous supportive blood product therapy utilizing packed red blood cells and platelets as appropriate. If appropriate chemotherapy can induce some degree of control of the tumor, improvement can on rare occasions occur.

Erythrocytosis (polycythemia)

Erythrocytosis or polycythemia can be seen as a manifestation of primary polycythemia vera or as a consequence of chronic hypoxia related to significant chronic pulmonary disease or significant right to left shunt due to congenital heart disease. Rarely an abnormal hemoglobin characterized by an increased oxygen affinity can be the cause of an erythrocytosis [43]. An elevated hematocrit and hemoglobin should be evaluated if necessary by a Cr^{51} blood volume to verify a genuine increase in red cells mass. An arterial blood gas is rarely necessary to confirm hypoxia. Polycythemia vera will present usually with leukocytosis, thrombocytosis, and often splenomegaly (two thirds of patients) and an elevated leukocyte alkaline phosphatase (LAP). There is a definite but rare instance of erythrocytosis associated with a variety of tumors. The most frequent of these tumors are renal cell carcinoma [44], hepatocellular carcinoma [45], cerebellar hemangioblastomas [46] and benign uterine fibromata. The incidence of erythrocytosis is approximately 20% in patients with cerebellar hemangioblastomas and 10% in patients with renal tumors. Increased production of erythropoietin or a an erythropoietin-like protein [47–50] have been found in patients with a renal cell carcinoma. Removal of the primary tumor has decreased or normalized hormonal production and serum or urinary levels so that the erythropoietin-like activity almost certainly is of tumor origin.

References

1. Bateman LJT, Beard MEJ. 1976. Malignant disease. In: Haematologic Aspects of Systemic Disease. Israel MCG, Delamore IW (eds). Saunders, London, pp 131-161.
2. Doll DC, Weiss RB. 1985. Neoplasia and the erythron. J Clin Oncol 3:429-446.
3. Eichner ER. 1979. Splenic function: Normal, too much and little. Am J Med 66: 311-320.

12

4. Goldman JM, Nolasco I. 1983. The spleen in myeloproliferative disorders. Clin Haematol 12:505–516.
5. Christinsen BE, Jonsson V, Videback A. 1983. The spleen in lymphoproliferative disorders. Clin Haematol 12:517–533.
6. Lynch EC, Alfrey CP Jr. 1965. Histiocytic medullary reticulosis. Hemolytic anemia due to erythrophagocytosis by histiocytes. Ann Intern Med 63:666–671.
7. Jaffe ES, Costa I, Fauci AS et al. 1983. Malignant lymphoma and erythophagocytosis simulating malignant histiocytosis. Am J Med 75:741–749.
8. Scott RB, Robb Smith AHT. 1939. Histiocytic medullary reticulosis. Lancet 2:194–198.
9. Cartwright GE. 1966. The anemia of chronic disorders. Sem Hematol 3:351–373.
10. Cartweight GE, Lee GR. 1971. The anemia of chronic disease. Br J Haematol 21:147–152.
11. Hyman GA, Gelhorn A, Harray J. 1956. Studies of the anemia of disseminated malignant neoplastic disease. II. Study of the life span of the erythrocyte. Blood 11:618–631.
12. Douglas SW, Adamson JW. 1975. The anemia of chronic disorders: Studies of marrow regulation and iron metabolism. Blood 45:55–65.
13. Dumick N, Kalkami V, Howard D et al. 1983. Mechanisms of abnormal erythropoiesis in malignancy. Cancer 51:1101–1106.
14. Chanarin I. 1976. Investigation and management of megaloblastic anemia. Clin Haematol 5:747–763.
15. Krantz S. 1974. Pure red cell aplasia. N Engl J Med 291:345–350.
16. Krantz, S. 1976. Diagnosis and treatment of pure red cell aplasia. Med Clin North Am 60:945–958.
17. Hirst E, Robertson TE. 1967. The syndrome of thymoma and erythroblastopenic anemia – A review of 56 cases. Medicine 46:225–264.
18. Sieff C. 1983. Pure red cell aplasia. Br J Haematol 54:331–336.
19. Mitchell ABS, Pinn G, Pegrum GD. 1971. Pure red cell aplasia and carcinoma. Blood 37:594–597.
20. Slater LM, Schultz MJ, Armentrout SA. 1974. Remission of pure red cell aplasia associated with non thymic malignancy. Cancer 44:1879–1881.
21. Natelson EA, Lynch EC, Hettig RA, Alfrey CP. Jr. 1968. Histiocytic medullary reticulosis. Arch Intern Med 122:223–229.
22. Tseng A Jr, Coleman CN, Cox RS et al. 1984. The treatment of malignant histiocytosis. Blood 64:48–53.
23. Dacie JV. 1975. Autoimmune haemolytic anemia. Arch Intern Med 135:1293–1306.
24. Jones JE. 1973. Autoimmune disorders and malignant lymphoma. Cancer 31:1092–1098.
25. Worlledge SH. 1978. The interpretation of a positive direct antiglobulin test. Br J Haematol 38:157–162.
26. Sokol RJ, Hewitt S, Stamps BK. 1981. Autoimmune hemolytic anemia: An 18 year study of 865 cases referred to a regional transfusion center. Br Med J 282:2023–2027.
27. Kyle RA, Kiely JM, Stickney JM. 1959. Acquired hemolytic anemia in chronic lymphocytic leukemia and the lymphomas. Arch Intern Med 104:61–67.
28. Eisner E, Ley AB, Meyer K. 1967. Coombs-positive hemolytic anemia in Hodgkin's disease. Ann Intern Med 66:258–273.
29. Levine AM, Thornton P, Forman SJ et al. 1980. Positive Coombs test in Hodgkin's disease: Significance and implications. Blood 55:607–611.
30. Garraty G, Petz LD, Wallerstein RO, Fudenberg HH. 1974. Autoimmune hemolytic anemia in Hodgkin's disease associated with anti-I^t. Transfusion 14:226–231.
31. Crisp D, Pruzanski W. 1982. B-cell neoplasms with homogenous cold-reacting antibodies (cold agglutinin). Am J Med 72:915–922.
32. Pruzanski W, Shumak KH 1977. Biologic activity of cold reacting autoantibodies. N Engl J Med 297:578–592.

33. Brain MC. 1970. Microangiopathic hemolytic anemia. Ann Rev Med 21:133–144.
34. Lohrmann HP, Adam W, Heymer B, Kubanek A. 1973. Microangiopathic hemolytic anemia in metastatic carcinoma. Ann Intern Med 79:368–375.
35. Brain MC. 1972. Microangiopathic hemolytic anemia. Br J Haematol 23:45–52.
36. Antman KH, Skarin AT, Mayer RJ, Hargraves HK, Canellos GP. 1979. Microangiopathic hemolytic anemia and cancer: A review. Medicine 58:377–384.
37. Alpert LI, Benisch B. 1970. Hemangioendothelioma of the liver associated with micro-angiopathic hemolytic anemia. Report of four cases. Am J Med 48:624–628.
38. Davis S, Rambotti P, Grignoni F. 1985. Microangiopathic hemolytic anemia and pulmonary small cell carcinoma. Ann Intern Med 103:638.
39. Cantrell JE, Phillips TM, Schein PS. 1985. Carcinoma-associated hemolytic anemia syndrome: A complication of Mitomycin C chemotherapy. J Clin Oncol 3:723–734.
40. Price TM, Murgo AJ, Keveney JJ et al. 1985. Renal failure and hemolytic anemia associated with Mitomycin C. A case report. Cancer 55:51–56.
41. Clifford GO. 1966. The clinical significance of leucoerythroblastic anemia. Med Clin North Am 50:789–799.
42. Ellmen L. 1976. Bone marrow biopsy in the evaluation of lymphoma, carcinoma and granulomatous disorders. Am J Med 60:1–7.
43. Valentine WN, Hennessey TC, Lang E et al. 1968. Polycythemia, erythrocytosis, and erythemia. Ann Intern Med 69:587–606.
44. Daman A, Holub DA, Medicow MM et al. 1958. Polycythemia and renal carcinoma: Report of ten new cases, two with long standing hematologic remission following nephrectomy. Am J Med 25:182–197.
45. Tso SC, Hua ASP. 1974. Erythrocytosis in hepatocellular carcinoma. Br J Haematol 28:497–503.
46. Waldmann TA, Levin EH, Baldwin M. 1961. The association of polycythemia with a cerebellar hemangioblastoma. The production of an erythropoietin stimulating factor by the tumor. Am J Med 31:318–324.
47. Lipsett MB, Odell WD, Rosenberg E, Waldmann TA. 1964. Numoral syndromes associated with nonendocrine tumors. Ann Intern Med 61:733.
48. Adamson JW, Finch CA. 1968. Erythropoietin and the polycythemias. Ann. NY Acad Sci 149:560–568.
49. Waldmann TA, Rosse WF, Swann RI. 1968. The erythropoietin-stimulating factors produced by tumors. Ann NY Acad Sci 149:509–515.
50. Hammond A, Winnick A. 1974. Paraneoplastic erythrocytosis and ectopic erythropoietin. Ann NY Acad Sci 230:219–227.

2. Hematologic disorders associated with cancer: II. White blood cell disorders

JO-ANNE M. BESSETTE

Introduction

White blood cell disorders that occur in patients with cancer include both quantitative and qualitative abnormalities. Many of the abnormalities of the white blood cell compartment are relatively benign and do not require treatment. These disturbances frequently are poorly understood in terms of etiology, sometimes waxing and waning with the disease process itself. The various interactions between the cancer and the white blood cell compartment remain to be elucidated.

Quantitative abnormalities

Leukocytosis and leukemoid reactions

Leukocytosis, an elevation in the absolute peripheral blood leukocyte count, is a common abnormality in patients with cancer. This can occur as a secondary phenomenon or as in the case of a myeloproliferative disorder such as chronic granulocytic leukemia (CGL), it is due to a primary defect in the hematopoietic stem cell.

Leukemoid reactions are defined as leukocytosis associated with immaturity of the white cells, so that myeloblasts and promyelocytes are seen in the peripheral blood. This white cell immaturity, which may resemble leukemia, is due to causes such as viral infection, inflammatory reaction, or neoplasia. The total leukocyte count may reach 50,000 to 100,000 cells per mm^3 with levels in excess of 100,000 per mm^3 rarely reported. To differentiate between a leukemoid reaction and CGL, measurement of the enzyme leukocyte alkaline phosphatase (LAP score) can be useful. The LAP score is characteristically low to absent in most patients with CGL, but is markedly elevated in leukemoid reactions. In addition, at least 85% of patients with

Higby, DJ (ed), Issues in Supportive Care of Cancer Patients. ISBN 0-89838-816-3.
© *1986, Martinus Nijhoff Publishers, Boston. Printed in the Netherlands.*

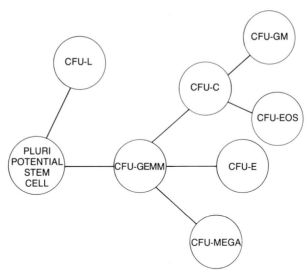

Figure 1. Hematopoietic development. (CFU-colony forming unit. L-lymphocyte. GEMM-granulocyte, erythroid, macrophage, monocyte. C-colony. GM-granulocyte monocyte. EOS-eosinophil. E-erythroid. MEGA-megakaryocyte).

CGL will have the Philadelphia chromosome, (PH_1 chromosome) while this chromosomal abnormality is absent in a leukemoid reaction.

The most frequent response to cancer is a mild to moderate leukocytosis composed primarily of mature polymorphonuclear neutrophils. All types of cancer, especially metastatic cancer, have been associated with leukocytosis, but lung cancer is the most common tumor described. The cause of leukocytosis is unknown but several mechanisms have been suggested including direct irritation or replacement of bone marrow by metastases, production of granulopoietic factor(s) by tumor tissue, or stimulation of the marrow by necrotic or infected tumor [1]. There are several studies using cell culture techniques that demonstrate the production of a granulopoietic factor called colony stimulating factor (CSF), by human lung cancers [2–6]. These are non small cell lung cancers with histologic types including squamous cell and large cell. Other tumors such as those arising from breast and ovary may also produce CSF [7, 8]. Polymorphonuclear leukocytes (granulocytes) are derived from progenitor cells in the bone marrow that have been stimulated to divide and grow by CSF. Figure 1 illustrates hematopoietic development from the pluripotential stem cell (capable of committment to any hematopoietic cell line) to the CFU-GM (the colony forming unit in *in vitro* culture that is committed to forming granulocytes and monocytes). Growth of CFU-GM requires CSF [9] which is composed of glycoproteins. It is thought that tumors may produce increased amounts of CSF, thus stimulating the growth of CFU-GM resulting in peripheral blood leukocytosis. There may be different types or concentrations of CSF that preferentially

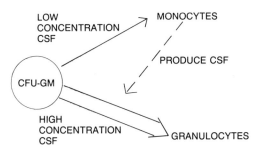

Figure 2. Rationale for the appearance of monocytosis before neutrophilia after drug-induced marrow suppression. As the primitive stem cell recovers, monocytic differentiation is possible with relatively low concentrations of colony stimulating factor (CSF). As monocytes increase in number, CSF is produced resulting in differentiation of CFU-GM to granulocytes.

promote growth of either granulocytes or monocytes. This may explain the appearance of neutrophilia in some patients and monocytosis in others.

Monocytosis

Monocytosis is frequently seen in patients with cancer. Monocytosis is defined as an increase in the absolute monocyte count greater than 500 per mm^3 in adults. In a series of 100 patients with known nonhematologic malignancies, over 60% had a monocytosis [10].

Monocytosis has also been seen in patients with lymphoma and Hodgkin's disease [11], in myeloproliferative disorders, in myelodysplastic syndromes particularly the category of chronic monocytic leukemia [12], and in histiocytic medullary reticulosis [13]. There is one report of a monocytic leukemoid reaction occurring in a patient with mediastinal teratoma and tuberculosis [14], but it is not clear whether the malignant disease was the cause since tuberculosis is also known to be associated with monocytosis.

Patients recovering from chemotherapy-induced bone marrow suppression sufficient to cause peripheral blood neutropenia will often exhibit a transient monocytosis, which heralds the recovery of the neutrophil count. It is felt that monocytes produce CSF necessary for granulopoiesis and since they may have the ability to grow at lower concentrations of CSF monocytes recover first and then produce the higher concentrations of CSF needed for neutrophil growth (Figure 2).

There is a report of an association between radiation therapy and monocytosis [15]. In this study of 29 patients with carcinomas including breast, lung, cervix, and prostate, there was a statistically significant increase in the absolute monocyte count during irradiation.

The significance of peripheral blood monocytosis in patients with cancer is not known. The essential role of the monocyte in immune surveillance, regulation of T lymphocyte function, and its ability to directly lyse tumor cells suggests that monocytosis may influence the course of the neoplasm. There are studies that suggest that infiltration of tumors by macrophages is associated with a more favorable prognosis in human cancers [16–18].

Eosinophilia

Eosinophilia, the elevation of the absolute eosinophil count to greater than 450 cells per mm^3, although more commonly seen in allergy and parasitic infections, is also associated with cancer. It has been frequently associated with Hodgkin's disease and mycosis fungoides, less commonly with other non-Hodgkin's lymphomas, and with acute lymphoblastic leukemia.

Tumor-associated eosinophilia has been divided into two categories: local tissue eosinophilia and peripheral blood eosinophilia [19]. Local tissue eosinophilia is usually associated with a good prognosis. Cervical cancer is the most common tumor associated with tissue eosinophilia. Others include lung cancer (squamous cell and large cell undifferentiated), and adenocarcinomas of the gastrointestinal or genitourinary tracts. Peripheral blood eosinophilia occurs in the late stages of cancer, usually in patients with extensive metastatic disease, and thus appears to be a poor prognostic sign. Peripheral blood eosinophilia occurs with the tumor types listed above as well as with carcinomas of the kidney, adrenal gland, thyroid, heart, and liver.

The eosinophil count may become markedly elevated. One patient with large cell carcinoma of the lung initially presented with a WBC of 9,400 with 12% eosinophils. The eosinophilia disappeared after surgical resection of the lung tumor. One year later with the development of diffuse metastatic disease the WBC rose to 161,000 with 78% eosinophils. The bone marrow showed no evidence of tumor but did show eosinophilic hyperplasia with 44% mature eosinophils [20].

It is possible that patients with marked eosinophilia secondary to cancer will develop organ damage (especially pulmonary) and cardiac disease from eosinophilic infiltration similar to that resulting from the hypereosinophilic syndrome. Some patients have been treated with steroids with a subsequent decrease in eosinophilia and improvement in symptoms, although the underlying malignancy continued to progress [21].

The cause of eosinophilia in cancer has been variously attributed to: (a) tumor necrosis with release of substances that attract eosinophils such as eosinophil chemotatic factor, ECF; (b) bone marrow metastases with consequent stimulation of eosinophil production; (c) tumor production of ECF or a CSF that promotes eosinophil production in the bone marrow, EOS-CSF.

Large cell carcinoma and anaplastic squamous cell carcinoma of the lung, as well as histiocytic lymphoma have been shown to produce ECF or EOS-CSF [22–24].

Eosinophilia has been reported following radiation therapy [25]. It may occur more commonly with abdominal irradiation and the suggestion has been made that radiation injury of dividing gastrointestinal cells is chemotactic for eosinophils and may stimulate their release and production.

Basophilia

Basophilia as a reaction to cancer is very rare, although it is commonly associated with CGL and other myeloproliferative disorders. An increase in the number of circulating basophils in CGL is usually a poor prognostic indicator since it heralds the onset of the accelerated phase of CGL or blastic transformation resulting in acute leukemia of either myeloid or lymphoid lineage. Rarely patients with CGL will develop a marked increase in the total WBC count with primarily basophils in the circulation, e.g. 'basophilic' leukemia. This can be associated with a hyperhistaminemic syndrome secondary to histamine release from the basophilia [26].

Lymphocytosis

Lymphocytosis is defined as an increase in the absolute lymphocyte count greater than 4,000 per mm^3 in adults. Lymphocytosis as a reaction to cancer is very rare. When present it resembles chronic lymphocytic leukemia (CLL) with over 50% mature lymphocytes. Previously described cases may have represented either a reaction to cancer or co-existent CLL. Surface marker analysis of the peripheral blood lymphocytes might be helpful in distinguishing these entities since in reactive lymphocytosis a polyclonal B lymphocyte population would be present, versus the monoclonal B lymphocyte population seen in most cases of CLL. A minority of cases of CLL are composed of T lymphocytes and perhaps even natural killer cells (NK cells) [27]. NK cells are thought to be a subset of T lymphocytes that morphologically resemble large granular lymphocytes and are capable of directly killing tumor cells [28]. The proliferation of NK cells might be a secondary event representing a response to an underlying chronic infection, chronic inflammation, or neoplasm [29]. In a case report of a patient with lymphocytosis and malignant fibrous histiocytoma, surgical removal of the tumor resulted in resolution of the lymphocytosis [30].

Plasmacytosis

Reactive plasmacytosis is characterized by an increase in the number of plasma cells (usually mature in appearance) in the bone marrow. This can occur secondary to infections, autoimmune disease, diabetes mellitus, liver cirrhosis, and neoplasia including Hodgkin's disease and acute myelogenous leukemia [31]. Reactive plasmacytosis is usually characterized by a polyclonal proliferation of plasma cells rather than the monoclonal plasma cell population that comprises multiple myeloma and Waldenstrom's macroglobulinemia. However, monoclonal gammopathy of undetermined significance (MGUS syndrome) is characterized by the expansion of a single cell clone as is seen in multiple myeloma with the expression of a monoclonal serum protein or M-component (an electrophoretically homogeneous immunoglobulin component), but most of these patients have a benign course [32].

The presence of a monoclonal serum protein has been detected in patients with lymphoproliferative disorders as well as solid tumors arising from colon, breast, prostate, lung, and stomach [33]. Reactive plasmacytosis in patients with cancer may be an immunological response to a tumor antigen.

Leukopenia

Leukopenia may occur as a result of the pancytopenia seen with marrow metastases with tumor cells replacing normal hematopoietic elements. It can occur as a result of splenic sequestration in those cancers associated with splenomegaly, especially myeloproliferative and lymphoproliferative disorders. Most commonly leukopenia in patients with cancer occurs as a result of chemotherapy and/or radiation therapy. The degree of cytopenia induced depends on multiple factors which affect the cellularity of the bone marrow. These include:

(i) age of the patient; younger patients have more cellular marrow with less fat and are more tolerant of a given drug dose than the elderly;

(ii) bone marrow reserve, which can be diminished by fibrosis, tumor involvement, previous chemotherapy and/or irradiation. Patients with diminished bone marrow reserve will be predisposed to develop cytopenias.

Because peripheral leukocytes have a short half-life (several hours) compared to platelets (7–9 days) and red cells (120 days), drug-induced myelosuppression results in leukopenia first, followed by thrombocytopenia. Generally the leukopenia is more severe than thrombocytopenia. This myelosuppression is usually reversible [34].

A decrease in the normal white blood cell count in leukemic states is thought to occur from neoplastic infiltration of marrow but also by the action of inhibitory factors that suppress the proliferation of normal white cells, giving the leukemic cells a survival advantage. This inhibitory activity has been demonstrated in bone marrow, spleen, and blood cells from patients with acute and chronic myeloid and lymphoid leukemia, lymphoma and preleukemia. It is thought that this inhibitory activity results from normal regulatory cell products that are overproduced in leukemia.

Leukemia-associated inhibitor (LAI) is released in leukemia by an unidentified but probably non-leukemic cell, and binds to normal CFU-GM, blocking the production of granulocytes and monocytes. Leukemic CFU-GM are not affected by LAI, perhaps because they lack receptors. A second type of inhibitory activity has been described called leukemia inhibitory activity (LIA) which differs from LAI. It has been characterized as an acidic isoferritin produced by monocytes and is thought to be a normal feedback regulator of granulopoiesis that prevents excessive white cell proliferation. Leukemia CFU-GM are insensitive to the effects of LIA [35–37].

Qualitative abnormalities

Neutrophil function

Chemotherapy, in addition to causing neutropenia, can also impair the function of white cells. Adriamycin has been shown to severely impair the phagocytic function of polymorphonuclear leukocytes in *in vitro* studies [38]. The peripheral blood neutrophils of breast cancer patients treated with combination chemotherapy regimens including cyclophosphamide, methotrexate, 5-flourouracil, vincristine, and prednisone, have been shown to have decreased phagocytic function [39]. Steroids can suppress the phagocytic function of granulocytes or monocytes by stabilizing lysosomal membranes.

Monocyte function

Abnormalities of monocyte function in cancer patients have been reported and include impaired phagocytosis [40], impaired chemotaxis [41, 42], impaired spontaneous monocyte-mediated cytotoxicity [43], and defective maturation [40]. There may be a correlation between the histologic grade and/or total body burden of the tumor with the presence of impaired monocyte function. In a study of patients with squamous cell carcinoma of the head and neck, the chemotactic responsiveness of monocytes was much more affected in those with poorly differentiated histologies than in those with well differentiated tumors [44].

Tumors may produce substances that impair monocyte function and in this way escape immune surveillance and the tumoricidal effect of activated monocytes [42].

Immune defects

Cancer can be associated with acquired immunodeficiency either through chemotherapeutic drugs that impair lymphocyte and/or monocyte function or as a consequence of the cancer itself. Patients with chronic lymphocytic leukemia can develop hypogammaglobulinemia and impaired cell-mediated immunity. In multiple myeloma there is a decrease in normal immunoglobulin levels. In Hodgkin's disease there is an increased incidence of abnormalities in cell mediated immunity, although the production of antibodies or humoral immunity is usually normal or over reactive [45]. Decreased numbers of peripheral blood T lymphocytes have been described in patients with cancer [46]. There are variable reports of changes in T lymphocyte subpopulations with either decreased numbers of T helper cells or increased numbers of T suppressor cells proposed as the cause of immunodeficiency [47, 48].

Studies are ongoing to determine the mechanism(s) of these immunologic abnormalities in patients with cancer. These may include the production of blocking or inhibitory factors by the tumor, hyperreactivity of the immune system in response to chronic antigenic stimulation (exposure to tumor antigen) possibly with eventual depletion of immune cells, or the activation of suppressor cells that inhibit the immune response.

References

1. Robinson WA. 1974. Granulocytosis in neoplasia. Ann NY Acad Sci 230:212–218.
2. Sato N et al. 1979. Granulocytosis and colony-stimulating activity (CSA) produced by a human squamous cell carcinoma. Cancer 43:605–610.
3. Suda T et al. 1980. A case of lung cancer associated with granulocytosis and production of colony-stimulating activity by the tumor. Br J Cancer 41:980–984.
4. Kimura N, Niho Y, Yanase T. 1982. A high level of colony-stimulating activity in a lung cancer patient with extensive leukocytosis, and the establishment of a CSA procucing cell line (KONT). Scand J Haematol 28:417–424.
5. Bockman RS, Bellin A, Repo MA, Hickok NJ, Kameya T. 1983. *In vivo* and *in vitro* biological activities of two human cell lines derived from anaplastic lung cancers. Cancer Res 43:4571–4576.
6. Okabe T et al. 1984. Establishment of a human colony-stimulating factor-producing cell line from an undifferentiated large cell carcinoma of the lung. Cancer 54:1024–1029.
7. Lee MA, Lottsfeldt JL. 1984. Augmentation of neutrophilic granulocyte progenitors in the bone marrow of mice with tumor induced neutrophilia: Cytochemical study of *in vitro* colonies. Blood 64:499–506.

8. Takeda A et al. 1904. Clear cell carcinoma of the ovary with colony-stimulating-factor production. Cancer 54:1019–1023.
9. Burgess AW, Metcalf D. 1980. The nature and action of granulocyte-macrophage colony-stimulating factors. Blood 56:947–958.
10. Barrett O. 1970. Monocytosis in malignant disease. Ann Intern Med 73:991–992.
11. Kaplan HS. 1980. Hodgkin's disease, second edition. Harvard University press, Cambridge MA.
12. Zittoun R. 1976. Subacute and chronic myelomonocytic leukemia: a distinct haematologic entity. Br J Haematol 32:1–5.
13. Warnke RA, Kim H, Dorfman RF. 1975. Malignant histiocytosis (histiocytic medullary reticulosis); Clinicopathalogic study of 29 cases. Cancer 35:215–230.
14. Gibson A. 1946. Monocytic leukemoid reaction associated with tuberculosis and a mediastinal teratoma. J Pathol Bacteriol 58:469–474.
15. Rotman M, Ansley H, Togow L, Stowe S. 1977. Monocytosis a new observation during radiotherapy. Int. J Rad Oncol Biol Phys 2:117–121.
16. Underwood JCE. 1974. Lymphoreticular infiltration in human tumors: prognositc and biological implications: a review. Br J Cancer 30:538–548.
17. Lauder I, Aherne W, Stewart J, Sainsbury R. 1977. Macrophage infiltration of breast tumors: a prospective study. J Clin Pathol 30:563–568.
18. Luebbers EL et al. 1977. Heterogeneity and prognostic significance of breast tumors: A prospective study. J Clin Pathol 30:563–568.
19. Lowe D, Jorizzo J, Hutt MSR. 1981. Tumor-associated eosinophilia; a review. J Clin Pathol. 34:1343–1348.
20. Kodama T et al. 1984. Large cell carcinoma of the lung associated with marked eosinophilia. Cancer 54:2313–2317.
21. Reddy Sethu KS, Hyland RH, Alison RE, Sturgeon JFG, Hutcheon MA. 1984. Tumor-associated peripheral eosinophilia: two unusual cases. J. Clin Oncol 2:1165–1169.
22. Goetzl EJ et al. 1978. Production of a low molecular weight eosinophil polymorphonuclear leukocyte chemotactic factor by anaplastic squamous cell carcinoma of human lung. J Clin Invest 61:770–780.
23. Wasserman S et al. 1979. Tumor associated eosinophilotactic factor. N Engl J Med 290:420–424.
24. Goetzl EJ et al. 1980. A novel eosinophil chemotactic factor derived from a histiocytic lymphoma of the central nervous system. Clin Exp Immunol 40:249–255.
25. Muggia EM, Ghossein NA, Wohl H. 1973. Eosinophilia following radiation therapy. Oncology 27:118–127.
26. Rosenthal S, Schwartz JH, Canellos GP. 1977. Basophilia chronic granulocytic leukemia with hyperhistaminaemia. Br J Haematol 36:367–372.
27. Pandolfi F et al. 1984. Classification of patients with T cell chronic lymphocytic leukemia and expansion of granulai lymphocytes: heterogeneity of Italian cases by a multiparameter analysis. J Clin Immunol 4:174–184.
28. Lotzova E. 1984. The role of natural killer cells in immune surveillance against malignancies. Cancer Bull 36:215–225.
29. Semenzato G et al. 1984. Abnormal expansions of polyclonal large to small size granular lymphocytes: reactive or neoplastic process? Blood 63:1271–1278.
30. Taylor HG, Terebelo HR, Gameza. 1982. Lymphocytosis in a patient with malignant fibrous histiocytoma. Cancer 50:1563–1567.
31. Gavarotti P, Boccadara M, Redoglia V, Golzio F, Pileri A. 1985. Reactive plasmacytosis. Case report and review of the literature. Acta Haematol 73:108–110.
32. Kyle RA. 1978. Monoclonal gammapathies of undetermined significance: natural history of 241 cases. Am J Med 64:814–826.

33. Isobe T, Osserman EF. 1975. Pathologic conditions associated with plasma cell dyscrasias: a study of 806 cases. Ann NY Acad Sci 190:507–512.
34. Hoagland HC. 1982. Hematologic complications of cancer chemotherapy. Sem Oncol 9:95–101.
35. Olofsson T, Olsson I. 1980. Biochemical characterization of a leukemia-associated inhibitor (LAI) suppressing normal granulopoiesis in vitro. Blood 55:983–991.
36. Bognacki J, Broxmeyer HE, Lobue J: 1981. Isolation and biochemical characterization of leukemia-associated inhibitory activity that suppresses colony and cluster formation of cells. Biochem. Biophys. Acta 672:176–190.
37. Olsson I, Olofsson T. 1985. Production characteristics and mode of action of hemopoietic growth inhibitors in myeloid leukemias (editorial). Med. Oncol Tumor Pharmacother 2:1–6.
38. Vaudaux P et al. 1984. Adriamycin impairs phagocytic function and induces morphologic alterations in human neutrophils. Cancer 54:400–410.
39. Matamoros MC, Walker BK, Van Dyke K, Van Dyke CJ. 1983. Effect of cancer chemotherapeutic agents on the chemiluminescence of human granulocytes. Pharmacol 27:29–39.
40. Samak R, Edelstein R, Bogucki D, Samak M, Israel L. 1980. Testing the monocyte-macrophage system in human cancer. Biomedicine 32:165–169.
41. Boetchu DA, Leonard EJ. 1974. Abnormal monocyte chemotactic response in cancer patients. J Natl Cancer Inst 52:1091–1099.
42. Snyderman R, Pike MC. 1976. An inhibitor of macrophage chemotaxis produced by neoplasms. Science 192:370–372.
43. DeYoung NJ, Gill PG. 1984. Monocyte antibody-dependent cellular cytotoxicity in cancer patients. Cancer Immunol. Immunother 18:54–58.
44. Balm FAJM et al. 1984. Monocuclear phagocyte function in head and neck cancer. Cancer 54:1010–1015.
45. Romagnani S, Ferrini PLR, Ricci M. 1985. The immune derangement in Hodgkin's disease. Sem Hematol 22:41–55.
46. Watanobe T et al. 1985. T cell subsets in patients with gastric cancer. Oncology 42:89–91.
47. Hayashi Y et al. 1984. Peripheral T gamma lymphocyte population in head and neck cancer. Cancer Immunol. Immunother 17:160–164.
48. McCluskey DR, Roy AD, Abram WP, Martin WMC. 1983. T Lymphocyte subsets in the peripheral blood of patients with benign and malignant breast disease. Br J Cancer 47:307–309.

3. Hematologic disorders associated with cancer: III. Coagulation disorders associated with neoplastic disease

RICHARD H. STEINGART

Introduction

Hemorrhagic, thrombotic and embolic complications occur frequently in cancer patients. Diverse hemostatic alterations including impaired plasma coagulation, platelet abnormalities and vascular disorders account for these defects. Not only have these defects been ascribed to an effect of the malignancy, but in fact the entire sequence of cancer cell growth and metastasis is intimately entwined with the hemostatic system.

In 1878, Billroth reported autopsy observations that human tumor cells were frequently found in association with thrombi. He went on to suggest that metastases occur when a portion of the tumor-thrombus complex breaks off and forms a tumor embolus [1]. This has been substantiated more recently in many experimental animal models [2]. It is thought that the clot can secure the firm arrest of cancer cells and lead to their diapedesis through the capillary wall and into tissues where they can become origins of metastatic foci. Plasminogen activators, enzymes commonly produced by malignant cell lines, produce proteolytic products of plasminogen and fibrinogen that may enhance local vascular permeability [3]. Platelet derived prostaglandins and growth factors may also influence tumor cell proliferation [4]. If tumors are dependant on fibrin deposition for their local spread, one might expect that inhibition of fibrinolysis would be associated with rapid spread of tumors; indeed, in rats, inhibition of fibrinolysis with epsilon aminocaproic acid has been shown to enhance tumor growth [5].

Until recently, human studies of defibrinating agents, anticoagulants, or fibrinolytic drugs in cancer have been limited to uncontrolled trials in heterogeneous groups of patients. However, the Veterans Administration Cooperative Study on the use of warfarin in the treatment of small cell carcinoma of the lung revealed that the median survival of patients who received warfarin in addition to standard chemotherapy (50 weeks) was significantly greater than the median survival of subjects who received chemotherapy

Higby, DJ (ed), Issues in Supportive Care of Cancer Patients. ISBN 0-89838-816-3.
© *1986, Martinus Nijhoff Publishers, Boston. Printed in the Netherlands.*

alone (26 weeks) [6]. The median length of time to evidence of tumor progression was also increased significantly in the warfarin group. Although this is suggestive evidence to support Billroth's hypothesis, the small size of the study and the possible tumoricidal effects of warfarin demand caution in interpreting the results. Heparin and antiplatelet agents have been less extensively studied and equivocal results have been reported to date [7].

Intravascular coagulation and fibrinolysis

Hypercoagulability and thrombosis

The association between malignancy and thrombosis has been recognized since 1865, when Trousseau described the syndrome of recurrent migratory thrombophebitis in a series of patients with gastric carcinoma [8]. Since then, a number of clinical and post mortem studies appeared describing arterial and venous thrombosis, migratory thrombophlebitis, pulmonary embolism and non-bacterial thrombotic endocarditis [9]. The overall incidence of thrombosis in patients with malignancies is between 5 and 15% [10]. The incidence of thromboembolic disease in post mortem studies of cancer patients is considerably higher [11]. Thromboembolic events rank second only to infections as causes of death in patients with solid tumors. Although patients with mucin-secreting tumors of the gastrointestinal tract have long been known to be prone to thromboembolic complications, other tumor types are also associated with an increased risk of thromboembolic disease. Pancreatic carcinoma has historically been associated with the greatest risk of thrombosis reported to be as high as 50% [12]. However, since the prevalence of lung cancer far exceeds pancreatic tumors the presence of thrombosis is most likely to be associated with tumors of the lung than of the upper gastrointestinal tract. The other more common tumors associated with thrombosis include gastric, colon, prostate, ovarian, breast and renal in descending order [9].

The incidence of thrombotic complications seen with specific tumor types are changing constantly due to chemotherapy and hormonal therapy. A recent series of 433 patients with breast cancer treated with chemotherapy, was reported in which the incidence rate of thromboembolic disease detected clinically was 5%. After chemotherapy was completed, no patients developed thrombotic complications [13]. Similarly, prostatic carcinoma has not been associated with a significantly increased risk of thromboembolic disease de novo. However, such patients appear to be at increased risk when treated with either chemotherapy or estrogen [14]. Surgical procedures also increase the risk of thrombotic events in patients with cancer compared to patients with non-malignant conditions [15].

Episodes of thrombosis, particularly superficial thrombophlebitis, may actually, antedate by months or even years, the clinical diagnosis of cancer in many patients [16]. However, the indications for conducting an extensive search for an occult malignancy in patients with deep vein thrombophelitis or pulmonary embolism are more vague. Cancer has been detected up to 2 years after the diagnosis of pulmonary embolism in 15% of patients [17].

Non-bacterial thrombotic endocarditis has been described primarily with adenocarcinoma of the lung, pancreas and colon. The most frequently involved valve is the aortic followed by the mitral valve. The larger the vegetation, the higher the frequency of embolization. The spleen is the most commonly infarcted viscus. However, end organs associated with greatest morbidity and mortality included cerebral vessels, coronary arteries and the renal bed.

The increased incidence of thromboembolic disease has led several investigators to examine various aspects of the coagulation system in patients with cancer. Subclinical coagulopathy is frequent in patients with malignancy. Abnormalities of routine tests of blood coagulation have been reported to occur in as many as 98% of patients with cancer [19]. The most common clotting abnormalities in cancer patients are elevated concentrations of fibrin split products (FSP), prolonged thrombin times, thrombocytosis and hyperfibrinogenemia. Other common abnormalities include decreased anti-thrombin III levels (AT III) and elevation of plasma coagulation factors including factors V, VIII, IX and XI [10]. These abnormalities have been said to be consistent with the presence of 'overcompensated intravascular coagulation with secondary fibrinolysis'. In this situation, it is theorized that low-grade intravascular coagulation with accelerated clotting factor utilization is accompanied by increased synthetic rates for fibrinogen, clotting factors, and platelets, resulting in actual increases in their levels in the circulation and a realtive hypercoagulable state.

Fibrinopeptide A (FPA) is a peptide that is cleaved from fibrinogen selectively by thrombin [20]. The increased FPA levels correlate with fibrinogen turnover rates in cancer patients, this providing further evidence that fibrin generation occurs at an increased rate. Rickles has demonstrated elevated levels of FPA in 60% of patients with solid tumors who had no evidence of thrombosis [21]. An upward trend of FPA correlated with progression of disease. Persistent elevation of FPA levels in individual patients suggested treatment failure and poor prognosis. On the other hand, in patients who entered remission, initially high levels of FPA trended towards normal.

The mechanism by which malignant tissue initiates disseminated intravascular coagulation (DIC) is poorly understood. Rickles and Edwards recently reviewed the evidence for three basic mechanisms for the activation of blood coagulation in patients with neoplastic disorders: (1) the activation of platelets by tumor cells; (2) the production of procoagulants by monocytes and macrophages, stimulated by tumor the tissue procoagulants antigens; (3) the production of procoagulants directly by tumor cells [7]. The tissue procoagulants derived from extracts of human breast, colon, kidney and lung cancer can directly initiate coagulation by activation of factor X to Xa [7, 22]. This differs from the conventional method of activation by thromboplastic substances via factor XII or factor VII.

The treatment of thromboembolic complications in patients with cancer is difficult. No controlled studies show superiority of one treatment approach over the other. However, it does appear that success in controlling the coagulopathy ultimately requires successful control of the underlying disorder. When laboratory abnormalities are found in the absence of clinical complications, treatment of the coagulopathy is generally not indicated. One exception is when subclinical DIC complicates acute promyelocytic leukemia (to be discussed later). The use of anticoagulants (warfarin, heparin) and antiplatelet drugs (salicylates, dipyridamole) have been associated with some correction of altered coagulation factors and clinical improvement. In spite of this, cancer patients are notoriously resistant to anticoagulation therapy and re-thrombosis is common [16].

In their review of chronic DIC in malignancy, Sack et al. found positive responses to anticoagulant therapy in 65 % of 55 patients when heparin was used initially, and 33 % of 26 patients treated with heparin after failing warfarin therapy. In contrast, only 19 % of 32 patients treated with warfarin alone responded [9]. Recurrent thromboembolic disease, especially in the setting of stable or increasing tumor burden, usually requires continued heparin therapy for a prolonged period. Once control of acute symptoms is achieved, outpatient management with subcutaneous heparin is often successful. Patients who do not respond to heparin therapy initially may be treated with antiplatelet agents. These may be as effective as heparin, and associated with less bleeding from tumor surfaces [10].

Hemorrhage

Intravascular coagulation is present in many patients with cancer and manifests varying clinical patterns, the most extreme form being acute DIC and fulminant catastrophic hemorrhage. The occurrence of overt DIC, characterized by consumption of platelets and clotting factors with resultant bleeding complications, is less common with solid tumors than is 'chronic' DIC manifested by thrombosis. Although acute DIC has been reported in association with almost all types of solid tumors, it is most commonly observed with carcinomas of the lung, gallbladder, stomach, colon, breast, ovary and melanoma [9, 10]. It is especially common in both local and metastatic carcinoma of the prostate. The incidence in different series range from 6 to 40 %. The neoplastic disorder most frequently associated with fulmitant DIC is acute promyelocytic leukemia.

Hemorrhagic complications in affected patients with solid tumors may range from minor mucocutaneous bleeding to extensive gastrointestinal, genitourinary, pulmonary or intracerebral hemorrhage. Patients with acute decompensated DIC will commonly manifest thrombocytopenia, hypofibrinogenemia, prolonged thrombin times, PT, PTT and elevated levels of circulating FSP. AT III as well as other clotting factors levels are usually reduced due to consumption. Less commonly, the peripheral blood smear will show evidence of microangiopathic red cell fragmentation.

Unlike the 'chronic' hypercoagulable form of this entity, in 'acute' DIC clotting factors are consumed in excess of production. The mechanisms by which tumors can cause any form of DIC has been discussed. The reason some tumors tend to favor clot formation and other clot lysis is not clear. However, in the case of prostate carcinoma, the neoplastic tissue contains procoagulant-like materials which can trigger both the extrinsic coagulation system as well the fibrinolytic system. This may explain why from a laboratory and clinical standpoint, the patient more often presents with bleeding. Acute promyelocytic leukemia is frequently associated with DIC. In many instances, subclinical DIC is converted to fulminant DIC with the initiation of cytotoxic chemotherapy. This is attributed to the release of a thromboplastin like material localized to the nuclear membrane and granules within the cells [23].

Therapy in the acute DIC of neoplastic disease should be initially directed at treatment of the underlying malignancy itself. Until antineoplastic therapy is initiated, control of bleeding is often unsuccessful. The first line of therapy for active bleeding often consistents of treatment with replacement products such as platelets and clotting factors. A major controversy exists concerning heparin usage. Although anticoagulant therapy has a clearer benefit with respect to chronic, as opposed to acute DIC, no randomized trials of heparin therapy in the DIC of malignancy have been conducted. Most recommendations are that if heparin therapy is to be used, it should be considered in acute DIC syndromes other than those associated with an acute treatable event such as sepsis.

In addition, heparin should be used cautiously, if at all, in the setting of severe renal or hepatic failure, when extensive vascular damage is present, or when very severe thrombocytopenia and hypofibrinogenemia are found. Despite the controversy regarding the use of heparin, Drapkin et al., in a non-randomized trials, compared 15 patients with acute promyelocytic leukemia treated between 1970 and 1975 with nine patients treated between 1975 and 1976; the first group received chemotherapy alone, while the second received chemotherapy and prophylactic heparin therapy [24]. In the heparin-treated group there was a decreased incidence of fatal hemorrhage and therefore an increased incidence of remission induction.

The doses of heparin used in the literature range from 300 to 600 U/kg/24 h. Continuous heparin infusion is preferable, since this mode of delivery is associated with fewer bleeding complications than pulse doses of heparin. For control of minor hemorrhagic complications such as recurrent epistaxis and gingival bleeding not associated with severe thrombocytopenia, some authors have advocated an initial trial of low-dose heparin (2500–5000 U subcutaneously 2–3 times a day) [10].

Primary fibrin(ogen)olysis

Primary fibrin(ogen)olysis is a hemostatic disorder in which there is either local or systemic activation of the fibrinolytic pathway resulting in plasmin degradation of fibrinogen, fibrin, factor V and factor VIII. Hypofibrinogenemia, very high circulating levels of FSP, low plasminogen levels, relatively normal levels of platelets and a very short englobulin clot lysis time should be present.

Although primary hyperfibrinolysis occurs in malignancy, DIC with secondary fibrinolysis is a much more common cause of hemorrhage. The more common tumors that are capable of spontaneous fibrinolytic activity include prostate carcinoma and sarcomas [25, 26]. In addition, Davidson et al. described a patient with metastatic large cell carcinoma of the lung whose tumor produced plasminogen activators that caused bleeding at the site of a surgical incision [27].

Distinction from a co-existing DIC syndrome may be difficult, but must be made before treatment with an inhibitor of plasminogen activation such as epsilon aminocaproic acid is considered. These drugs can cause severe thrombotic complications in the setting of DIC [28].

Other coagulation defects

Patients with neoplastic disease may develop bleeding from other coagulation factor abnormalities. These are less common and are usually associated with less serious hemorrhage than when DIC develops. Hepatic dysfunction, due to neoplastic parenchymal damage or to obstruction of the biliary system, may produce a variety of coagulation defects. Reduced synthesis and poor absorption of vitamin K may lead to deficiencies, in particular, of the vitamin K dependent factors (II, VII, IX and X). Vitamin K supplementation is usually ineffective and hemorrhage must be controlled with fresh frozen plasma. Factor XIII is the precursor of an enzyme that induces covalent cross-linkage between fibrin monomers, producing tensile strength to the clot. Factor XIII deficiency or dysfunction may be seen in metastatic liver disease and may result in poor wound healing [29]. Because of the long half-life of factor XIII (4–7 days) and the small amounts required to achieve normal hemostasis, this deficiency is easily corrected with relatively infrequent administration of fresh frozen plasma. Of particular significance, although rare, is the development of a dysfibrinogenemia in association with hepatocellular carcinoma or less commonly with other cancers metastatic to the liver [30, 31]. Bleeding tends to be mild and usually occurs from the mucous membranes. Hemostasis can be obtained by the use of either fresh frozen plasma or cryoprecipitate. Since the half-like of infused fibrinogen is 4–6 days, replacement may be necessary only once or twice a week.

Isolated deficiencies of individual coagulation factors are rare, and for the most part, the etiology of the acquired deficiency state is unknown. Most have only mild decreases in factors and are therefore clinically asymptomatic. Philadelphia chromosome positive chronic myelogenous leukemia has been associated with deficiencies of factor XII, factor XIII and factor V [32–34]. Of interest, the factor V level has been observed to normalize after cytoreduction in some patients. Factor XI deficiency has been described in one patient with metastatic melanoma [35]. Certain deficiencies may be associated with clinical bleeding. A hemorrhagic disorder secondary to adsorption of factor VIII procoagulant and factor VIII related antigen by lymphocytes has been described in a patient with Waldenstrom's macroglobulinemia [36]. The same abnormalities, suggestive of acquired Von Willebrand's disease, have also been noted in patients with chronic lymphocytic leukemia, poorly differentiated lymphocytic lymphoma and Wilm's tumor [37–39]. In all cases, the clotting abnormality corrected after remission was obtained. Amyloidosis has been associated with an acquired deficiency of factor X. Levels range from 1 to 20 %. Approximately two-thirds of patients have some hemorrhagic disorder [40]. The mechanism appears to be due to binding of factor X to the amyloid fibrils [41]. The deficiency of factor X is corrected poorly, if at all, by transfusion of plasma or activated factors. Griepp, et al., have demonstrated that removal of a large spleen infiltrated with amyloid can relieve the factor X deficiency [42].

The vast majority of acquired circulating anticoagulants are antibodies either neutralizing a specific blood coagulation factor or interfering in some fashion with factor interactions. Inhibitors may occur with a wide variety of tumors. They are usually more significant clinically in paraproteinemias than in solid tumors. Anticoagulant activity in paraproteinemias have been demonstrated against factor VIII, VII, V and prothrombin [40]. IgG paraproteins are usually directed against factor prothrombin or factor VII, while IgA and IgM paraproteins are directed against factor VIII and factor V [43]. Coagulation inhibitors with heparin-like activity have also been described in multiple myeloma [44, 45]. The most common coagulation paraprotein interaction appears to be inhibition of fibrin monomer polymerization. It appears that paraprotein selectively attacks the fibrin monomer and impedes polymerization into a stable fibrin clot [40]. Abnormalities in both the thrombin time and reptilase time are reliable indicators of this defect. As might be expected, response of the plasma cell dyscrasia to chemotherapy is often accompanied by improvement in the hemostatic abnormalities. In addition, plasmapheresis may temporarily lead to rapid correction of the abnormal hemostatic parameters [46].

Lupus anticoagulants are best defined as inhibitors that interfere to a variable degree with phospholipid dependant coagulation tests without inhibiting activity of any specific coagulation factor. They have been identified in a few patients with Hodgkin's disease, non-Hodgkin's lymphoma, myelofibrosis and carcinoma [47–49]. When present as isolated abnormalities, these are not associated with a bleeding disorder; in fact, hypercoagulability has been seen [50]. Inhibitors to factor XI have been detected in patients with carcinoma of the colon and prostate [25, 52]. A circulating anticoagulant to factor VII has been described in a patient with carcinoma of the lung [52].

Platelet abnormalities

Thrombocytopenia

Thrombocytopenia is the most common cause of bleeding in patients with both solid tumors and hematologic malignancies. Decreased production of platelets can result from systemic chemotherapy, radiotherapy or direct invasion of the marrow with tumor. The degree of thrombocytopenia usually correlates well with the degree of marrow infiltration [53]. The bone marrow biopsy is much more reliable than the aspirate to detect bone marrow involvement by carcinoma [54]. Ineffective thrombopoiesis, characterized by dysplastic or megaloblastic marrow, hypercellularity and peripheral cytopenia is usually caused by sepsis, B12 or folate deficiency, or primary myelodysplastic syndromes. Correction of the underlying infection or nutritional deficiency may result in improved counts. Platelet counts of less than $10,000 \text{ mm}^{-3}$ are often association with spontaneous hemorrhage and therefore most advise support with platelet concentrates. An ideal platelet concentrate contains approximately 1×10^{11} platelets and, in general, one unit of platelet concentrate will elevate the platelet count by $5000–7000 \text{ mm}^{-3}$. Spontaneous bleeding with platelet counts greater than $50,000 \text{ mm}^{-3}$ is rare. With counts between $20,000 \text{ mm}^{-3}$ and $50,000 \text{ mm}^{-3}$ bleeding is usually associated with traumatic or surgical stress.

Thrombocytopenia due to increased peripheral destruction most commonly indicates the presence of DIC, hypersplenism, or an autoimmune phenomenon. A syndrome resembling idiopathic thrombocytopenic purpura (ITP) is most often associated with lymphoproliferative malignancies. Case reports of patients with non-small cell and small cell lung cancer, as well as adenocarcinomas of the rectum, colon, ovary and gallbladder have been described as having ITP-like syndromes [55]. These may develop prior to, concident with, or following the diagnosis of cancer. The diagnosis is established by finding thrombocytopenia with adequate to increased number of megakaryocytes in the marrow without evidence of DIC, drug-induced thrombocytopenia, or myelopthesis. Platelet associated antibody testing has been found to be very sensitive but not very specific in patients with ITP. Therefore it is not routinely used as a diagnostic test. Several patients with solid tumors and ITP syndrome were found to have both IgG and IgM platelet specific antibody [56]. Response of platelet counts to high-dose (60 mg/day) prednisone is common but transient. However, 60% of patients may obtain a complete response to splenectomy [55]. Very rarely, increased platelet destruction due to thrombotic thrombocytopenic purpura may occur with malignancy [57, 88].

Thrombocytosis

Thrombocytosis is said to occur in up to 30 to 40% of cancer patients. It is more often associated with carcinomas but has been described in both Hodgkins and non-Hodgkins lymphomas. The etiology may be due to increased thrombopoietic activity [7]. The platelet count is usually modest, ranging from $400,000 \text{ mm}^{-3}$ to $800,000 \text{ mm}^{-3}$. The platelets appear morphologically normal. Clinical bleeding or thrombosis from this isolated problem is rare. The differential diagnosis of thrombocytosis in the cancer patient includes myeloproliferative disorders; acute and chronic inflammatory disorders; acute hemorrhage; iron deficiency; hemolytic anemia; an asplenic state (usually surgical); or a response to vincristine or epinephrine. As of now, no specific treatment of the thrombocytosis is indicated except to treat the underlying malignancy. Treatment of thrombocytosis is ordinary required only in the myeloproliferative disorders when the platelet count exceeds $1,000,000 \text{ mm}^{-3}$ and there is clinical evidence of thrombosis or hemorrhage.

Qualitative platelet disorders

Abnormal platelet function is common in both solid tumors and hematologic malignancies. In solid tumors, the most common cause of defective platelet function is the presence of FSPs resulting from DIC or fibrinolysis. Additional platelet abnormalities have also been noted. These include decreased platelet factor 3 and a decreased aggregation response to ADP [58]. The clinical significance of these platelet defects is not established.

Hemorrhagic manifestations frequently occur in the dysproteinemias, where abnormalities of platelet function much more commonly account for clinical bleeding than do thrombocytopenia or factor deficiencies. The actual incidence of hemorrhage in malignant paraprotein disorders varies depending upon the particular disease. About 15% of patients with IgG myeloma and over 38% with IgA myeloma experience bleeding. Patients with Waldenstrom's macroglobulinemia have a greater than 60% incidence of hemorrhage [59]. Impaired *in vitro* platelet function is attributed to coating of the platelet canalicular system with paraprotein [60]. This abnormality is acquired by normal platelets incubated in dysproteinemic plasma. Hemostatic and laboratory abnormalities are related to the concentration of paraprotein [59]. Several specific platelet defects have been described. These include decreased platelet retention by a glass bead filter, impaired platelet aggregation, and decreased platelet factor 3 availability [59, 61, 62]. It is of interest that some individuals demonstrate abnormal platelet aggregation and adhesion, but have normal bleeding times and the absence of clinical bleeding. Treatment of hemorrhage is directed towards decreasing the paraprotein by either chemotherapy or, more acutely, with plasmapheresis [63]. Other causes of acquired qualitative platelet defects in patients with cancer include uremia, liver disease, and the use of certain B-lactam antibiotics [64].

Vascular disorders

Neoplastic diseases of the endothelium may result in purpuric and hemorrhagic lesions. Chief among these is Kaposi's sarcoma. Once primarily a disease of older Italian and Jewish men, this disease has become increasingly more common and noticeable due to its association with acquired immune deficiency syndrome (AIDS). The cell of origin in this disease appears to be the endothelial cell [66]. Preliminary therapeutic trials suggest that the 'epidemic' forms of Kaposi's sarcoma are responsive to several agents including Vinblastine, VP-16, interferon and immunoabsorption [66–69]. Using vincristine boluses, Mintzer has reported several responses of Kaposi's sarcoma associated with thrombocytopenia in patients with AIDS [70].

Amyloid deposits occur in the area between the endothelium and the basement membrane, thereby infiltrating the subendothelium in both the microcirculation and macrocirculation. The infiltrated vessel has decreased tensile strength and constriction abilities. Extravastion, including purpura, may occur [71]. Purpura may be one of the presenting signs in as many as 16% of all patients with amyloidosis [72]. The distribution of the lesion has a peculiar prediliction for the face.

In malignant dysproteinemic states, such as multiple myeloma and Waldenstrom's macroglobulinemia, purpuric lesions may result from associated cryoglobulinemia or cryofibrinogenemia. Cryofibrinogens have also been noted in patient with metastatic malignancies [73]. Histologically, leukocytoplastic vasculitis is noted and constituents of the cryoglobulin may be demonstrable. Therapy has included steroids, plasmapheresis and treatment of the underlying disease.

Purpura is frequently seen in Cushing syndrome. It may be seen in patients who have received glucocorticoids for extended periods. This type of purpura is typically superficial and limited to the forearms. Glucocorticoids decrease collagen synthesis and may result in reduction of structural support for the microcirculation [74].

Effects of chemotherapy on hemostasis

Chemotherapy may alter hemostasis by a variety of mechanisms. The most common and significant of these have been previously discussed and include the thrombocytopenia associated with bone marrow suppressive cytotoxic drugs and the enhancement of DIC by drug-induced destruction of some malignant neoplasms.

L-Asparaginase cytotoxicity results from inhibition of protein synthesis. Nearly 100% of patients develop hypofibrinogenemia in the absence of DIC. Depression of factors IX and XI has been noted in a majority of patients. Although laboratory studies suggest a severe coagulopathy, clinical bleeding is rare. Upon discontinuance of therapy, the coagulation parameters correct in about 7 days [75].

Mithramycin may cause severe thrombocytopenia. However, 50% of bleeding episodes occur in patients with platelet counts greater than 100,000 mm^{-3}. Although some studies describe depression of coagulation factors II, V, VII and X, this is not a consistent finding [76, 77]. More often a reversible qualitative platelet disorder is found, characterized by prolongation of the bleeding time associated with decreased platelet aggregation responses to ADP, collagen and epinephrine [77].

The use of doxorubicin and daunorubicin have been associated with activation of the fibrinolytic system and subsequent clinical hemorrhage [78, 79]. L-phenylalanine mustard has also been reported to cause qualitative platelet dysfunction [80]. The clinical significance remains unclear.

References

1. Billroth T. 1878. Lectures on surgical pathology and therapeutics (translated from the 8th edition). The New Sydenham Society.
2. Chew E, Wallace AC. 1976. Demonstration of fibrin in early stages of experimantal metastasis. Cancer Res 36:1904–1909.
3. Peterson HI. 1977. Fibrinolysis and antifibrinolytic drugs in the growth and spread of tumors. Cancer Treat Rep 1:213–217.
4. Ross R, Voge A. 1978. The platelet derived growth factor: Review. Cell 14:203–210.
5. Cliffton EE, Agostino VMD. 1964. Effect of inhibitors of fibrinolytic enzymes on development of pulmonary metastasis. J Natl Cancer Inst 33:753–763.
6. Zacharski LR, Henderson WG, Rickles FR et al. 1981. Effect of warfarin on survival in small cell carcinoma of the lung. JAMA 245:831–835.
7. Rickles FR, Edwards RL. 1983. Activation of blood coagulation in cancer: Trousseau's syndrome revisited. Blood 62:14–31.
8. Trousseau A. 1865. Phlegmasia alba dolens. Clinique Medicale de l'Hotel-dieu de Paris, London. New Sydenham Society 3:94.
9. Sack GH, Levin J, Bell W. 1977. Trousseau's syndrome and other manifestations of chronic disseminated coagulopathy in patients with neoplasms. Clinical, pathologic and therapeutic features. Medicine 56:1–37.
10. Bick RL. 1978. Alterations of hemostasis with malignancy. Sem Thromb. Hemost 5:1–26.
11. Ambrus JL, Ambrus CM, Mink IB et al. 1975. Causes of death in cancer patients. J Med 6:61–64.
12. Ambrus JL, Ambrus CM, Pickern J et al. 1975. Hematologic changes and thromboembolic complications in neoplastic disease and their relationship to metastasis. J Med 6:433–458.
13. Weiss RB, Toriney DC, Holland JF et al. 1981. Venous thrombosis during multimodal treatment of primary breast carcinoma. Cancer Treat Rep 65:677–679.
14. Kasimis BS, Spiers AS. 1979. Thrombotic complications in patients with advanced prostatic cancer treated with chemotherapy. Lancet 1:159.
15. Pineo GF, Brain MC, Galkes AS et al. 1974. Tumors, mucus production and hypercoagulability. Ann NY Acad Sci 230:262–270.
16. Schafer AI. 1985. The hypercoagulable states. Ann. Intern Med 102:814–828.
17. Gore JM, Appelbaum JS, Greene HL et al. 1982. Occult cancer in patients with acute pulmonary embolism. Ann Intern Med 96:556–560.
18. Rohner RF, Prior JT, Sipple JH. 1966. Mucinous malignancies, venous thrombosis and terminal endocarditis with emboli. Cancer 19:1805–1812.
19. Sun NC, McAfee WM, Gibert JM et al. 1979. Hemostatic abnormalities in malignancy, a prospective study of one hundred eight patients. Am J Clin Path 71:10–16.
20. Peusher FW, Cleton FJ, Armstrong L et al. 1980. Significance of plasma fibrinopeptide A (fpA) in patients with malignancy. J Lab Clin Med 96:5–14.
21. Rickles FR, Edwards RL, Baub C et al. 1983. Abnormalities of blood coagulation in patients with cancer. Cancer 51:301–307.
22. Pineo GF, Regorezi F, Hatton MWC. 1973. The activation of coagulation by extracts of mucin: a possible pathway of intravascular coagulation accompanying adenocarcinomas. J Lab Clin Med 82:255–260.
23. Gralnick HR, Sultan C. 1975. Acute promyelocytic leukemia: Haemorrhagic manifestation and morphologic criteria. Br J Haematol 29:373–376.
24. Drapkin RI, Gee TS, Dowling MD et al. 1978. Prophylactic heparin therapy in acute promyelocytic leukemia. Cancer 41:2484–2490.

25. Goldsmith GH Jr. 1984. Hemostatic disorders associated with neoplasia. In: Disorders of Hemostasis. Ratnoff OD, Forbes CD, (eds). Grune & Stratton, Orlando, pp 351–363.

26. Cliffon EC, Grossi CE. 1955. Fibrinolytic activity of human tumors as measured by the fibrinplate method. Cancer 8:1146–1147.

27. Davidson JF, McNicol GP, Frank GC. 1969. Plasminogen-activator producing tumor. Br. Med J 1:88–91.

28. Rachmilewitz EA. 1967. Defibrination syndrome followed by hypercoagulable state. Thromb Daith Haemorh 17:120–128.

29. Soong BC, Miller sp. 1970. Coagulation disorders in cancer III. Fibrinolysis and inhibitors. Cancer 25:867–874.

30. Felten A, Straub RW, Frick PD. 1969. Dysfibrinogemia in a patient with primary hepatoma. First observation of an acquired abnormality in fibrin momomer aggregation. N. Engl J Med 280:405–409.

31. Green G, Thomson JM, Dymock IW et al. 1976. Abnormal fibrin polymerization in liver disease. Br J Haematol 34:427–439.

32. McGrath K, Koutts J. 1975. A case of Hageman factor deficiency with myeloid leukemia. Aust NE J Med 5:155–157.

33. Rasche Dietrich M, Gaus W et al. 1974. Factor XIII-activity and fibin subunit structure in acute leukemia. Biomed 21:61–66.

34. Haseqawa DIC, Bennett AJ, Coccia PF et al. 1980. Factor V deficiency in Philadelphia-positive chronic myelogenous leukemia. Blood 56:585–595.

35. Phillips JP, O'Shea MJ. 1977. A new coagulation defect associated with a case of melanomatosis. J Clin Path 30:547–550.

36. Brody JI, Haidar MD, Rossman RE. 1979. A hemorrhagic syndrome in Waldenstrom's macroglobinemia secondary to immunoadsorption of factor VIII. N Engl J Med 300:408–410.

37. Wautier JL, Levy-Toledano S, Caen JP. 1976. Acquired von Willebrand's syndrome and thrombopathy in a patient with chronic lymphocytic leukemia. Scand j Haematol 16:128–134.

38. Joist JH, Cowein JF, Zimmerman TS. 1978. Acquired von Willebrand's disease. N Engl J Med 298:988–991.

39. Noronha PA, Hruby MA, Maurer HS. 1979. Acquired von Willebrand disease in a patient with Wilm's tumor. J Peds 95:997–999.

40. Shapiro SS, Hultin M. 1975. Acquired inhibitors to the blood coagulation factors. Sem Thromb Hemostat 1:336–351.

41. Furie B, Voo L, Kieth PW. 1981. Mechanism of factor X deficiency in sytemic amyloidosis. N Engl J Med 304:827–830.

42. Greipp PR, Kyle RA, Bowie EW. 1979. Factor X deficiency in primary amyloidosis: resolution after splenectomy. N Engl J Med 301:1050–1051.

43. Lackner H. 1973. Hemostatic abnormalities associated with dysproteinemias. Sem Hematol 10:125–133.

44. Palmer RN, Rick ME, Rick PD. 1984. Circulating heparin sulfate anticoagulant in a patient with a fatal bleeding disorder. N Engl J Med 310:1696–1699.

45. Khoory MS, Nesheim ME, Bowie W. 1980. Circulating heparin sulfate proteoglycan anticoagulant from a patient with a plasma cell disorder. J Clin Invest 65:666–673.

46. Perkins HA, McKenzie MR, Fudenberg HH. 1970. Hemostatic defects in dysproteinemias. Blood 35:695–707.

47. Goldsmith GH, Saito H, Muir WA. 1981. Labile anticoagulant in a patient with lymphoma. Am J Hematol 10:305–311.

48. Scleider MA, Nachman RL, Jaffe EA et al. 1976. A clinical study of the lupus anticoagulant. Blood 48:499–509.

38

49. Yanq HC, Kuzur M. 1977. Procoagulant specificity of factor VIII inhibitor. Br J Haematol 37:429–433.
50. Mueh JR, Herbst KD, Rapaport SI. 1980. Thrombosis in patients with lupus anticoagulants. Ann Intern Med 92:156–159.
51. Criel A, Collen D, Masson PL. 1978. A case of IgM antibodies which inhibit the contact activation of blood coagulation. Thromb Res 12:883–892.
52. Campbell EB, Sanal S, Mattson J et al. 1980. Factor VII inhibitor. Am J Med 68:962–964.
53. Slickter SJ, Harker LA. 1974. Hemostasis in malignancy. Ann NY Acad Sci 230:252–261.
54. Ingle JN, Tormey DC, Tan HK. 1978. The bone marrow examination in breast cancer. Cancer 41:67–674.
55. Kim HD, Boggs DR. 1979. A syndrome resembling idiopathic thrombocytopenia purpura in 10 patients with diverse forms of cancer. Am J Med 67:371–276.
56. Bellone JD, Kunnicki TH, Asrer RH. 1983. Immune thrombocytopenia associated with carcinoma. Ann Intern Med 99:470–472.
57. Brook J, Konwaler BE. 1965. Thrombotic thrombcytopenic purpura. Association with metastatic gastric carcinoma and a possible autoimmune disorder. Calif Med 102:222–227.
58. Friedman IA, Schwartz so, Leifhold SL. 1964. platelet function defects with bleeding. Arch Intern Med 113:177–185.
59. Perkins HA, Mackenzie MR, Fudenberg HH. 1970. Hemostatic defects in dysproteinemias. Blood 35:695–707.
60. Pachter MR, Johnson SA, Neblett TR et al. 1959. Bleeding, platelets and macroglobulinemia. Am J Clin Pathol 31:467–482.
61. Saraya AK, Kasturi J, Kishan R. 1972. A study in hemostasis in macroglobulinemia. Acta Haematol 47:33–42.
62. Penny R, Castaldi Pa, Whitsed HM. 1971. Inflammation and haemostasis in paraproteinemias. Br J Haematol 20:35–44.
63. Lacker H. 1973. Hemostatic abnormalities associated with dysproteinemias. Sem. Hematol 10:125–133.
64. Brown CH, Bradshaw MW, Natelson EA et al. 1976. Defective platelet function following the administration of penicillin compounds. Blood 47:949–956.
65. Burgdorf W, Mukal K, Rosai J. 1979. Immunohistochemical identification of factor VIII in endothelial cells of normal skin and in cutaneous lesions of alleged vascular nature. Clin Res 27:523A.
66. Lewis B, Abrams D, Ziegler J et al. 1983. Single agent or combination chemotherapy of Kaposi's sarcoma in acquired immune deficiency sydrome. (Abstract) Pro Am Soc Clin Oncol 2:59.
67. Laubenstein LJ, Krigel RL, Hymes KB et al. 1983. Treatment of epidemic Kaposi's sarcoma with vp-16-213 and a combination of doxorubicin, bleomycin and vinblastine. (Abstract) Pro Am Soc Clin Oncol 2:228.
68. Groopman JE, Gottlieb MS, Goodman J et al. 1984. Recombinant alpha-2 interferon therapy for Kaposi's sarcoma associated with the acquired immunodeficiency syndrome. Ann Intern Med 100:671–676.
69. Peters W. 1985. Personal communication.
70. Mintzer DM, Real FX, Jouino L. 1985. Treatment of kaposi's sarcoma and thrombocytopenia with vincristine in patients with the acquired immunodeficiency syndrome. Ann Intern Med 102:200–202.
71. Kitchens CS. 1984. The purpuric disorders. Sem Thromb Hemostat 10:173–189.
72. Kyle RA, Bayrd ED. 1975. Amyloidosis. Review of 236 cases. Medicine (Baltimore) 54:271–299.

73. Zlotnick A, Shahin W, Rachmilewltz EA. 1969. Studies in cryofibrinogenemia. Acta Haematol 42:8–17.
74. Prockop DJ, Kiuirikko KI. 1967. Hydroxyproline and the metabolism of collagen. In: Biology of collagen vol 2 of treatise on collagenld. Gould S (ed).Academic Press, London, p 230.
75. Ramsay NIC, Coccia PF, Kriuit W et al. 1977. The effect of L-asparaginase on plasma coagulation factors in acute lymphoblastic leukemia. Cancer 40:1398–1401.
76. Monto RW, Talley RW, Caldwell MJ. 1969. Observations on the mechanisms of hemorrhagic toxicity in mithramycin therapy. Cancer Res 29:697–703.
77. Ahr DJ, Scialla SJ, Kimball DB. 1978. Acquired platelet dysfunction following mithramycin therapy. Cancer 41:448–454.
78. Bick RL, Fekete WF, Wilson WL. 1976. Adriamycin and fibrinolysis. Thromb. Res 8:467–475.
79. Bick RL, Feket L, Murano G. 1976. Daunamycin and fibrinolysis. Thromb Res 9:201–203.
80. Klener P, Kubisz P, Suranova J. 1977. Influence of cytotoxic drugs on platelet functions and coagulation. Thromb Haemostat 37:53–61.

4. Defense mechanisms and infections in cancer patients

GERALD J. ELFENBEIN

Introduction

The goals of this chapter are to discuss the principles of normal host defense mechanisms against infectious diseases, to describe the clinical circumstances in which host defense mechanisms break down in cancer patients, and to give some examples of the types of infectious processes which may occur in the secondary compromised state related to malignancies. This chapter is not intended to be an exhaustive review of the literature nor an encyclopedia of infectious diseases in cancer patients. Rather, its object is to discuss how host defense mechanisms normally reduce susceptibility to infectious diseases. By understanding the relationships of host defense mechanisms and specific infectious processes, it is possible to devise prophylactic and therapeutic maneuvers to reduce the morbidity and mortality from some infectious diseases in cancer patients. One other disclaimer: this chapter will not deal with the defense mechanisms against nor the infectious processes caused by multicellular parasites and most unicellular parasites (with the exceptions of *Pneumocystis carinii* and *Toxoplasma gondii*).

Host antimicrobial defense mechanisms

The primary functions of the immune system are tolerance to self antigens (prevention of autoimmune disorders), resistance to infections, tolerance of the fetal allograft (during pregnancy), regulation of stem cell differentiation for myelopoiesis and lymphopoiesis, and surveillance against neoplasms. The immune system is, however, but one of the defense mechanisms that the host has to resist infections. As will be seen in this section, the immune system, albeit very sophisticated, is relegated to the position of being the third line of defense against primary infections.

Higby, DJ (ed), Issues in Supportive Care of Cancer Patients. ISBN 0-89838-816-3.
© *1986, Martinus Nijhoff Publishers, Boston. Printed in the Netherlands.*

Epithelial barriers and invasion

Perhaps one of the most important components of the host defense mechanisms against infectious disease is the epithelial barrier. The epithelial barrier is sometimes only one cell thick but its physical integrity and proper function is critical to resistance against infections. Epithelial barriers represent the interface between the host and the environment. Intact epithelial barriers resist invasion by microbes from the environment. Thus, the epithelium is the first line of defense against infections. The epithelial barriers include specifically the integument, the conjunctivae, the upper and lower respiratory epithelia, the mucosa of the gastrointestinal tract, the uroepithelia, and the epithelia of the genital tract.

Each epithelium has some special physical and functional properties which facilitate resistance against invasion by microbes. The integument is a multicellular, multilayered structure which presents a formidable mechanical barrier. In addition, the chemical properties (acid pH) of sebum secreted by the sebaceous glands reduce bacterial colonization that is well known to occur on the surface of the skin and especially in the skin appendages (hair follicles, sweat glands, etc.). The conjunctivae are constantly bathed by tears, which are produced by the lacrimal glands and which contain lysozyme that further defends against microbial invasion. The respiratory tract is coated by mucus which it secretes and which entraps microorganisms. The tracheo-bronchial tree has a ciliated columnar epithelium. The cilia tend to sweep microbes entrapped in mucus upward to the hypopharynx from which the mucus is swallowed. The oral cavity, pharynx and esophagus have multicellular, multilayered epithelia. Swallowing moves contents from these spaces into the stomach where the profound acidity and the proteolytic enzymes are usually effective in decontaminating what is swallowed. The small bowel is usually sterile if there is no obstruction to the flow of material being digested. The large bowel is usually colonized by gram negative and anaerobic bacteria. The unicellular columnar epithelaium secretes mucus and serves as a barrier to invasion by microbes. In addition, the colonizing organisms often produce bactericidal substances which are lethal to super-infecting bacteria which sometimes are considerably more pathogenic than the colonizing bacteria. Constant flow of a usually acid pH urine helps to protect the uroepithelium from even colonizing microbes. In the female genital tract, the pH and colonizing bacteria are important defense mechanisms of the vagina in addition to the multicellular, multilayered structure of the epithelium. The mucus plug in the os of the uterine cervix is also an effective barrier to microbial invasion.

The major principles responsible for effective resistance of epithelia to microbial invasion are thickness of the epithelium, constant flow of fluids across the epithelium (washing), production of secretions with entrapment and bactericidal properties, and the beneficial relationship with microorganisms (commensals) which normally colonize the epithelium. Interference with any of these may be sufficient to permit invasion across the epithelial barrier.

Phagocytic cell system

The second line of defense against invading microbes are the cells of the phagocytic system. These cells, upon encountering microbes either in the tissues or in the circulation, ingest and then kill the microbes with digestive enzymes contained in lysosomes. The phagocytic cell system is an 'immediate response' system. There are, basically, two compartments of the phagocytic cell system. They are the circulating phagocytes and the sessile reticuloendothelial system.

Circulating phagocytic cells

Circulating phagocytic cells are derived from hematopoietic stem cells. They are the polymorphonuclear leukocytes (polys) and monocytes. They are released from the sinusoids of the bone marrow into the circulation. Polys are terminally differentiated cells which lack capability to proliferate. On the other hand, monocytes do have the ability to differentiate in the tissues into tissue macrophages and, further, into multinucleated giant cells. Polys and monocytes spend a portion of their life span in the circulation. Most of their life span, however, is spent outside of the circulation in the extracellular fluid which bathes the tissues. Polys and monocytes exit from the circulation by diapedesis through the endothelial cells of capillaries.

In many regards polys and monocytes are ameboid and represent single cell defenders against microbes. When in the tissues beneath epithelia in the vicinity of invading microbes, polys and monocytes (depending on the type of microorganism) have the ability to phagocytose and lyse the invading microorganism. This process does not require any assistance but is greatly facilitated by the inflammatory response and by opsonins.

Inflammatory process

The inflammatory process is a local phenomenon probably initiated by the first interaction of phagocytes with microorganisms. (It may also be initiated by cell bound immunoglobulin with specificity for the microbe – see below.) This process involves vascular dilatation, leakage of fluid across the capillary membrane, and release of chemoattractants which recruit additional phagocytes from the circulation (chemotaxis) to the site of microbial invasion. There is a series of biochemical mediators (including activated complement components – see below) of the inflammatory response. The net effect is magnification of the number of phagocytes available to attach to and kill the invading microbes. Sometimes, the result is a pyogenic response which localizes the infection with massive accumulation of polys, results in necrosis of tissue and polys, and terminates in the formation of an abscess. Eventually, pus (polys and necrotic tissue) drains through tissue planes because of pressure necrosis. The acid pH and low oxygen tension of pus in the abscess further aid in killing invading microorganisms.

Opsonins

Opsonins are present in the circulation and extracellular fluids. Opsonins are molecules which attach to microbes and facilitate phagocytosis by polys. Some opsonins are nonimmune, i.e., nonspecific for the invading microbe, and others are immune, i.e., specific for the invading microbe. The alternate pathway of complement, i.e., the properidin system, provides nonimmune opsonins while immunoglobulins (see below) provide immune opsonins. During inflammation the leakage of fluid from the capillaries provides more opsonins which have the net effect of improving the efficiency of phagocytosis by polys.

Sessile reticuloendothelial system

The sessile reticuloendothelial system (RES) is also derived from hematopoietic stem cells, although the mechanism by which this occurs is not completely clear. Phagocytic cells of this system reside in the tissues. On the one hand, tissue histiocytes and alveolar macrophages appear to have some migratory properties and are not 'truly sessile'. These cells have the function of phagocytosing invading microorganisms whether they came by direct invasion or by inhalation. On the other hand, the 'truly sessile' phagocytic cells reside in the sinuses of the liver, spleen, bone marrow and lymph nodes. These cells have the function of clearing the blood and the lymph of invading microorganisms that have escaped from the local tissues into either the lymphatic or blood circulation. Much less is known about the mechanism of action of these 'filters' for the circulatory system than is known about polys and monocytes. However, blockage of the RES by noninfectious particulate materials reduces the ability of the RES to clear the circulation of microbes subsequently introduced.

From what has been described above, it is clear that deficiencies in quantities or dysfunctions of polys, monocytes, the inflammatory response, nonspecific opsonins, and the RES can permit an invading microorganism to establish a serious or life-threatening local or systemic infection.

Immune system

As stated above, the immune system is the third line of defense against

CYTOLYSIS OF VIRAL INFECTED CELLS

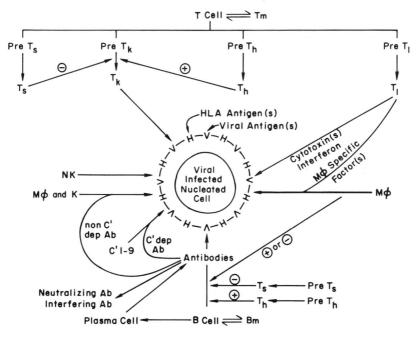

Figure 1. Schematic representation of potential effector mechanisms of the immune system attacking a virus infected human cell. Abbreviation used are: T_m = memory T cell; T_s = suppressor T cell; T_k = cytotoxic T cell; T_h = helper T cell; T_l = lymphokine producing T cell; NK = natural killer cell; MO = macrophage; K = lymphocyte mediating antibody dependent cellular cytotoxicity; C' = complement; dep = dependent; Ab = antibody; B_m = memory B cell.

invading microbes. It is relegated to this position because time (measured in weeks) is required upon first exposure to an invading microbe before an effective immune response can be generated. This is called the primary immune response. Upon second exposure to an invading microbe, the immune system works hand in hand with the phagocytic cell system in defending against invading microbes, some of which is mentioned in 'Phagocytic cell system' above. Also, upon second exposure there is a further, incremental generation of the effective immune response. This is called the secondary immune response. The secondary response is quicker (measured in days) than the primary response because of immunologic memory. The net effect of the secondary response is both an expansion of the immune response and an improvement in its ability to cope with the offending invading microbe.

Also as stated above, the immune system is highly sophisticated, very intricate, and carefully balanced by autoregulation. It is not possible to describe all of this in a limited space. An attempt to summarize the potential interactions of the immune system with a virus infected host cell (as a model for the action of the immune system) is shown in Figure 1. The rest of this section will deal with important principles of the immune system.

The immune system has, essentially, two compartments – a humoral compartment and a cellular compartment. In the humoral compartment are immunoglobulin molecules, complement components and cytokines. In the cellular compartment are B cells, T cells natural killer (NK) cells, K cells, and macrophages. The function of one set of these molecules and cells is highly antigen specific and requires prior exposure (i.e., immunization) before sufficient numbers of molecules (e.g., antibodies) and cells (e.g., killer T cells) are present for an effective immune response. The immune sytem has a remarkable ability to respond to a vast array of different antigens. This ability to respond to antigen diversity is now explained at the molecular biology level. Furthermore, the products of this immune response bind antigen avidly (i.e., they have a high affinity constant).

The function of a second set of molecules and cells is not antigen specific and does not require prior exposure or immunization before sufficient numbers of molecules (e.g., complement components) or cells (e.g., NK cells, K cells and macrophages) are present for an effective response. However, at least in the case of the complement components of the classical pathway and macrophages and K cells that can mediate antibody dependent cellular cytotoxicity, specific immunoglobulin reacting with specific antigen is required before activation of complement (by the classical pattern) or antibody dependent cellular cytotoxicity (by macrophages and K cells) occurs.

Finally, a third set of molecules and cells appears only after the interaction of T cells with specific antigen. By themselves, the molecules (e.g., interleukin-2 and gamma-interferon) and the cells (e.g., lymphokine activated killer cells and activated macrophages) are not antigen dependent in their activity; however, they appear to be extraordinarily important effectors of function of the immune system.

Were any of the components of the immune response to be depleted or defective, then this chink in the armor of the third line of defense could permit an invading microorganism to cause serious or life-threatening local or systemic infections.

The secondary compromised state

From the basic physiology discussed above, it can be seen that secondary compromise of the host can be produced by a breach in any of the epithelial barriers, a deficiency of any kind in the phagocytic cell system, and/or a defect of any type in the immune system. In fact, more than one defect or deficiency is usually seen in the cancer patient. In the secondary compromised state, these defects/deficiencies are produced by disease and/or therapy. They will be discussed in detail below. However, before defining the different kinds of defects/deficiencies seen under specific clinical circumstances, there are some important principles of the physiology of infectious microorganisms and their relationships with the host that must be explored in order to understand more fully the specific infectious diseases of the cancer patient.

Microorganism and other host factors conditioning infections

We have already discussed the notion that infectious disease in cancer patients is related to host permissiveness because of defective host defense mechanisms. This permissiveness does not itself produce infection; it merely permits infection to occur. There are two other important factors which determine whether and where specific infectious processes occur in cancer patients. They are the proximity of microorganisms to the host and a favorable milieu for replication of the microorganisms.

Proximity of microorganisms

No infection occurs if microorganisms are totally absent from the environment (both internal and external) of the host no matter how susceptible the host may be. This has been elegantly shown in germ-free animal models. However, cancer patients do not live in germ-free environments nor can they be rendered germ-free during therapy to prevent infectious diseases. Thus, we must consider the three situations in which microorganisms are proximate to the cancer patient and, thus, in appropriate location to cause infectious diseases. The three locations from which infections arise are the local external environment, surface colonization of epithelia, and latent endogenous microorganisms.

Local external environment

The local external environment is an important source from which infections may be acquired by the cancer patient. The local external environment places microorganisms in proximity to epithelial barriers. The local environment includes the air which patients breathe, food and water which patients consume, the water with which patients are bathed, and the medical team which takes care of the patient. Each of these can provide vectors of infection for the cancer patient. Examples are: airborne (*Aspergillus* spores), ingested (enteric pathogens), surface contaminants (gram negative pathogens), and transmitted by personnel (antibiotic-resistant *Staph. aureus* and *Enterobacter cloacae*).

Surface colonization of epithelial surfaces
In the real world, surface colonization of epithelial surfaces is an ordinary occurrence for the skin, upper respiratory passages, lower intestine, and female genital tract. Organisms that reside on these surfaces may be beneficial (commensals) or merely resident without known benefit. In any event, when epithelial barriers are disrupted, these organisms may gain entry to the tissues below the epithelial barrier and establish infections. When cancer patients are treated with antibiotics, the epithelial surfaces often become supercolonized by microorganisms that are resistant to antibiotics. In other words, the antibiotics disturb the normal flora colonizing epithelial surfaces. In the absence of normal flora, surfaces are supercolonized by organisms which are often more virulent and more pathogenic because of antibiotic resistance. Examples are: skin (antibiotic resistant *Staph. epidermidis* and *Corynebacterium* species) and large intestine (*Pseudomonas aeruginosa* and *Serratia marcescens*).

Latent endogenous microorganisms
Finally, reactivation of latent endogenous microorganisms is an important mechanism of infections for cancer patients. These organisms have already invaded and produced infections which have been clinically eradicated; however, microorganisms persist in the host without producing infection or inducing host defense mechanisms (e.g., the immune system) to respond to them. Latent infectious agents are usually located intracellularly.

The intracellular forms of latent microorganisms may be intact infectious agents (e.g., *Toxoplasma gondii*) or microbial genomes incorporated into host DNA (e.g., cytomegalovirus [CMV]). In any event, these latent microorganisms may be activated to produce infections in the cancer patients. Activation may be produced by disease and/or therapy. Examples of infectious processes which may be due to reactivation are: *Herpes simplex* types I and II, *Herpes zoster* virus, and toxoplasmosis.

Favorable milieu

Microorganisms have organ/tissue tropism. This means there are certain tissues or organs of the body where the sum total of biochemical properties provides a milieu most favorable for microorganism proliferation. In addition, there are other tissues or organs where the biochemical milieu is not favorable. Microorganisms find the milieu favorable to them by chance after direct invasion or by lymphatic or hematogenous spread. Proliferation of microorganisms is established at sites where the milieu is favorable. The specific requirements for proliferation of a particular microorganism are genetically determined. An example of this is reactivation pulmonary tuberculosis, which is almost always in the apical segments of the upper lobes where oxygen tension in the alveoli is the highest because *Mycobacterium tuberculosis* prefers high oxygen tension to proliferate.

In addition, there are host determined factors which condition the milieu and determine whether or not a tissue or organ is a favorable for proliferation of microorganisms. As a consequence of disease or as a toxicity of therapy the biochemistry of a tissue or organ can be altered such that the milieu is now favorable to proliferation of a microorganism. An example of this is CMV interstitial pneumonia after allogenic bone marrow transplantation for malignancies. CMV pneumonia is facilitated by both acute graft-versus-host disease and prior exposure of the lungs to irradiation during total body irradiation.

Clinical circumstances of the secondary compromised state

There is a wide variety of clinical circumstances associated with the secondary compromised state in the cancer patient as either a consequence of malignancy or therapy for malignancy or both. It is not possible in a limited space to catalogue all the clinical circumstances of the secondary compromised state which make the cancer patient susceptible to infectious diseases. A number of specific examples which illustrate the principles discussed above are given in Table 1. It must be remembered that most often more than one defect in host defense mechanisms is associated with specific malignancies and their therapy.

Disturbance of the epithelial barrier

As a consequence of disease or therapy an epithelial barrier to invasion may be disrupted. This means a physical break in the mechanical barrier to invasion. When this occurs surface microbes may easily pass into the underlying tissues. This is most often seen with the integument and gastrointestinal tract.

Even though the mechanical barrier to invasion may remain intact, the function of the epithelium may be sufficiently impaired to reduce resistance to microbial invasion. The epithelia which are particularly susceptible to impairment of function are the tracheobronchial tree (ciliary motion), the

Table 1. Examples of clinical circumstances and therapies which may produce a secondary compromised state in the cancer patient.

I.   Epithelial barriers
    A. Disrupted barrier
        1. Integument – tinea pedis, tinea cruris
        2. Gastrointestinal tract – mucosistis due to cytotoxic drugs and radiation
    B. Impaired function
        1. Ciliary motion of respiratory epithelium – alcoholism
        2. Continuous flow of fluid – ureteropelvic junction obstruction, small bowel dysmotility (blind loop syndromes following surgery)
        3. Secretion of tears by lacrimal glands – radiation therapy and Sjogren's syndrome
        4. Colonization of GI tract by candida – antibiotics
II. Phagocytic cell system
    A. Circulating phagocytes
        1. Deficient numbers
            a. Neutropenia – myelosuppressive therapy, rheumatic disorders
        2. Defective function
            a. Impaired poly phagocytosis – diabetes mellitus, alcoholism
II. B. Sessile RES
        1. Deficient tissue
            a. Splenectomy – Hodgkins disease
            b. Replacement – malignant reticuloendothelioses
III. Immune system
    A. Diminished immunoglobulins
        1. Increased loss – extensive hemorrhage
        2. Decreased production – multiple myeloma, corticosteroid therapy, bone marrow transplantation
    B. Diminished cellular immune responses
        1. Acquired loss – aging
        2. Endogenous suppression – Hodgkins disease, chronic graft vs. host disease after bone marrow transplantation
        3. Exogenous depression
            a. Diseases – protein malnutrition, lymphoid malignancies, CMV viral infection
            b. Therapies – corticosteroids, cytotoxic drugs, radiation therapy, antithymocyte globulin for acute graft vs. host disease
    C. Diminished cytokines
        1. Interleukin (1 and 2) production – bone marrow transplantation, chemotherapy for acute myelogenous leukemia

uroepithelium (drainage), and the gastrointestinal tract (propulsion). In addition, reduction of secretions and impairment of drainage of the conjunctiva and vagina, respectively, render these surfaces vulnerable to microbial supercolonization and potential invasion. Finally, with the pressure of antibiotics often used in the secondary compromised state, the normal flora which colonizes the skin and gastrointestinal tract is often replaced by flora which is more pathogenic because of antibiotic resistance as well as other intrinsic virulence properties of the microbes.

Impairment of the phagocytic cell system

There are basically two mechanisms whereby circulating phagocytes lose their efficacy in dealing with invading microbes. Circulating phagocytes may be present in insufficient numbers or, if present, their function may be impaired. Probably the most common cause of insufficient numbers of polys is cytotoxic, myelosuppressive therapy currently used for the treatment of cancer as well as in the immunosuppression necessary for organ (e.g., bone marrow) transplantation. Phagocytic function by polys may be impaired in diabetes mellitus and in alcoholism which may precede or develop after the diangosis of cancer.

Impairment of the reticuloendothelial system *per se* is not usually a cause for a secondary compromised state. However, it is now well recognized that 'debulking' the RES by splenectomy increases the risk of bacterial sepsis, which implies that the spleen is a major organ in host defenses against infections. Splenectomy is often performed during the staging of Hodgkins disease. From animal models it is clear that the RES can be blocked by intravenous injection of nonmetabolizable particles that are cleared from the circulation.

Depression of the immune system

Once primed, the immune system is very important in coping with invasive microorganisms for which epithelial barriers and phagocytic cells provide little protection for the host. When the immune system is impaired, these infections may become serious or life-threatening.

Immunoglobulins are antibody molecules with diverse specificities. Immunoglobulin levels may fall consequent to excessive loss or decreased production. It is theoretically possible to decrease immunoglobulins levels by increased catabolism but no clinical syndrome with this mechanism of immunoglobulin depletion is yet recognized.

The whole spectrum of cellular immune responses is susceptible to derangements that result in impaired function and, ultimately, increased susceptibility to infections. With age, cellular immune functions deteriorate. More commonly, and more often biologically significant, cellular immune responses are suppressed by clearly identifiable immunoregulatory cells (endogenous suppression) or depressed by clearly identifiable clinical syndromes or therapies (exogenous depression). No matter what mechanism is responsible for impairment of the immune system, the net result is increased susceptibility to infections, with resultant high morbidity and mortality.

Categorization of infections in cancer patients

It must by now be apparent that virtually any microorganism with any iota of virulence may infect a cancer patient in the secondary compromised state. In fact, the secondary compromised host is often the best 'culture medium' for infectious agents. Still, the infections which most often occur are those that would be most expected from our understanding of host defense mechanisms, microorganism factors, and other host factors described above. In this section, an attempt will be made to categorize the types of infections seen in cancer patients (see Table 2). Two basic categories are recognized – pyogenic organisms and opportunistic organisms.

Pyogenic organisms

Once epithelial barriers are deranged, pyogenic organisms may invade the tissues. Invasion of pyogenic organisms comes from colonizing (or supercolonizing) organisms or organisms acquired from the external environment. Because polymorphonuclear leukocytes, with the assistance of antibodies and complement, usually produce pus when combatting these organisms, they are referred to as 'pyogenic'. However, not all interactions of polys with these 'pyogenic' organisms result in pus formation even under normal circumstances.

Opportunistic organisms

The most serious type of infection in the secondary compromised host is produced by opportunistic organisms. Opportunistic organisms may be

Table 2. Examples of organisms which may infect concer patients.

I.   Pyogenic organisms – acquired and colonizing
    A.   Gram positive bacteria – *Staph. aureus, Staph. epidermidis, Corynebacterium* sp., Diphtheroids, *Strep. viridans, Strep. pneumoniae*
    B.   Gram negative bacteria – *H. influenza, N. meningitidis, Pseudomonas aeruginosa, Klebsiella-Enterobacter* sp., *E. Coli, Serratia marcescens*
    C.   Anaerobic bacteria – *Clostridia* sp., *Bacteroides* sp.
    D.   Fungi – *Candida albicans*
II. Opportunistic organisms – acquired, colonizing and reactivated
    A.   Bacteria – *Listeria monocytogenes, Mycobacteria* sp.
    B.   Fungi – *Candida* sp., *Torulopsis, Mucor* sp., *Aspergillus* sp.
    C.   Viruses – *H. simplex* (I and II), *H. Zoster,* cytomegalovirus
    D.   Protozoa – *Pneumocystis carinii, Toxoplasma gondii*
    E.   Others – legionella, mycoplasma, chlamydia

---

acquired from the environment, derived from colonization (or supercolonization), or derived from reactivation. They are called opportunistic organisms because in normal hosts they usually do not produce any infectious process, or produce limited infections. Control of these organisms and the infections they produce is a function of the immune system in healthy individuals. As can be seen from Table 2, opportunists may be bacterial, fungal, viral, or protozoal in nature. Ultimately, it is from epidemiologic studies that the specific infectious agents complicating specific clinical circumstances come to be well known.

Prophylaxis and therapy of infections in cancer patients

The principles of prophylaxis and therapy for the infections of cancer patients are derived from the principles of good practice for infectious diseases and from the principles we have described above.

Prophylaxis

The prevention of infections in cancer patients clearly depends upon the type of secondary compromise and the epidemiology of infectious diseases that occur under the specific clinical circumstances in question. It is well known that it is impossible to prevent all infections by a single or even a number of maneuvers. There is no clinical equivalent to the germ-free animal colony situation.

The principles of prophylaxis, then, take into consideration the epidemiology of the infections and the mechanisms by which the infections are normally handled. Every reasonable attempt should be made to avoid acquisition of pathogens from the external environment. Where appropriate, this may mean reverse isolation, laminar air flow rooms, carefully controlled diets, restrictions on number of visitors, restrictions on gifts (e.g., fresh flowers) for the patients, sterile water for bathing, hand washing by the medical team and visitors, and masks (on occasion). It is difficult, if not impossible, to sterilize all epithelial surfaces which are colonized by microorganisms. It may be best to try to keep epithelial barriers intact and, if this is not possible, to be prepared to treat the consequences of invasion by colonizing organisms. Broad spectrum antibiotics as prophylaxis are of limited value and potentially dangerous as they may reduce the normal flora and permit supercolonization with antibiotic-resistant and otherwise more virulent flora.

Until the mechanisms of reactivation of latent organisms are fully understood and alternatives in therapy for cancer are available, it will be impossible to prevent the reactivation of all latent organisms. It may, however, be possible to mute the clinical consequences or delay the reactivation of specific organisms with specific maneuvers. Chemoprophylaxis with acycloguanosine (acyclovir) is effective in bone marrow transplant recipients in delaying the reactivation of *H. simplex* types I and II. And, when simplex infections do occur in bone marrow transplant patients, they are less serious after acyclovir chemoprophylaxis. In addition, seroprophylaxis of CMV infections after bone marrow transplantation with immune globulin has been shown to mute the severity of CMV infections if not decrease the number of CMV infections after bone marrow transplantation. Thus, prevention of specific pathogens is possible provided there is effective, specific prophylaxis available.

Therapy

There is little new to say under the category of therapy for infections in cancer patients. Two principles are, however, worth enunciating. First, every possible effort should be made to identify *quickly* the specific pathogen producing the infections. Once identification is made by Gram stain, culture, or histopathology, the infection is treated with specific antibiotics. Second, if it is not possible to determine the pathogen or, if time does not permit, the patient must be treated with broad spectrum antibiotics with the intent of covering the most likely infectious agents based upon epidemiologic studies in the specific clinical circumstances in which the patient falls.

Conclusions

This chapter has made an attempt to present the principles of infectious diseases in cancer patients. It is important to understand the complexities of normal host defense mechanisms. It is important to understand the biology of the microorganisms and other host factors which condition infectious diseases. It is important to understand what host defense mechanisms are defective in each clinical circumstance (disease and/or therapy). And it is important to understand the epidemiology of infectious diseases in cancer patients. When all these are understood, it is possible to devise prophylactic strategies for some of the potential infections which may occur in cancer patients. If all infections were readily diagnosable and easily treatable without leaving significant residual deficits, then it would only be necessary to know how to diagnose and treat the infections of cancer patients. Unfortunately, this is currently not the case.

References

1. Davis BD, Dulbecco R, Eisen HN, Ginsberg HS (eds). 1980. Microbiology: Including Immunology and Molecular Genetics, 3rd Edition. Harper & Row, Philadelphia, PA.
2. Hoeprich PD (ed). 1980. Infectious Diseases: A Modern Treatise of Infectious Processes, 3rd Edition. Harper & Row, Philadelphia, PA.
3. Mandell GL, Douglas Jr RG, Bennett JE (eds). 1985. Principles and practice of Infectious Diseases, 2nd Edition. John Wiley & Sons, New York, NY.
4. Allen JC (ed). 1976. Infection and the Compromised Host. Williams & Wilkins, Baltimore, MD.
5. Allen JC (ed). 1981. Infection and the Compromised Host: Clinical Correlations and Therapeutic Approaches, 2nd Edition. Williams & Wilkins, Baltimore, MD.
6. Grieco MH (ed). 1980. Infections in the Abnormal Host. Yorke Medical Books, New York, NY.
7. Good RA (ed). 1984. Intravenous Immune Globulin and the compromised Host. Am J Med 76:Supplement 3A.

5. Regional chemotherapy

CHARLES F. WHITE and KAREN ANTMAN

Introduction

It is important to the supportive care of many cancer patients to deliver effective antineoplastic therapy selectively to regionally confined tumor. Even in the presence of widespread metastases, regional deposits of cancer often cause specific morbidity. Surgery and radiation therapy, classically considered 'local cancer therapy', frequently fail or are contraindicated. Regional chemotherapy in some cases represents the optimal treatment of regionally confined cancer, particularly for palliation.

This chapter will review the historical development and major indications for regionally administered chemotherapy. The rationale, pharmacology, and toxicology as well as a review of the anatomy and required techniques, will be stressed to help enable the oncologist to administer regional chemotherapy safely, intelligently and effectively. Ongoing and completed studies of regional chemotherapy studies will be summarized. The focus for future efforts will be discussed.

Rationale

Many chemotherapy agents are characterized by a steep dose response curve for both toxicity and therapeutic effect; that is, the higher the concentration, the greater the antitumor effect, and frequently, the more intense the side effects [1] (Figure 1). The ability to produce higher systemic drug levels is often limited by toxicity to normal host tissues, such as bone marrow and gastrointestinal mucosa. Administration of chemotherapy to a localized area is a potential means of increasing drug levels regionally while keeping systemic levels below toxic thresholds. Under favorable conditions, regional drug exposures may be increased 10- to 2000-fold over those achieved by equivalent doses given intravenously [2]. The two major methods of admin-

Higby, DJ (ed), Issues in Supportive Care of Cancer Patients. ISBN 0-89838-816-3.
© *1986, Martinus Nijhoff Publishers, Boston. Printed in the Netherlands.*

58

DOSE RESPONSE CURVE

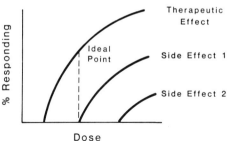

Figure 1. Dose response curve.

istering regional chemotherapy include infusion of drug into the arterial supply of the tumor (IA), and instillation of drugs into a third space compartment (cerebral spinal fluid, peritoneal, pleural, and pericardial cavities). Authors reviewing regional drug delivery range from pessimists who assert that the techniques are so complex that they are never worthwhile, to optimists convinced that direct drug delivery of higher drug levels to the tumor must be better than systemic delivery, regardless of the drug or the tumor site. Development of new devices such as totally implantable infusion pumps and access devices (Ommaya reservoirs, Infusaid pumps, Port-A-Caths(R), etc.) as well as an improved theoretical and practical understanding of regional chemotherapy pharmacokinetics and pharmacology [3] have stimulated renewed interest in regional chemotherapy.

Certain drugs possess properties making them attractive for regional delivery. Similarly, some sites of drug delivery are more favorable than others. This review will focus on sites and techniques where regional chemotherapy has been used most intensively.

Infusional chemotherapy

Regional chemotherapy was first reported in 1950, by C.T. Klopp who had delivered nitrogen mustard through the external carotid arteries for head and neck cancer [4]. While interest in this form of therapy has waxed and waned, interest has been rekindled recently because of technologic advances and a better understanding of drug pharmacokinetics. Intraarterial chemotherapy has been most extensively used to treat primary and metastatic cancer in the liver but has also been applied in head and neck cancer, brain tumors, extremity sarcomas, melanomas, and urogenital tumors. Successful intraarterial (IA) chemotherapy depends upon: (1) catheter placement to insure infusion of the entire tumor-bearing region; (2) use of a drug with appropriate pharmacokinetic and dose-response characteristics; and (3) a reliable, safe drug delivery system which preferably can be used by outpatients [2] (Table 1). The assumption underlying the use of intraarterial chemotherapy is that a higher concentration of a particular drug will be delivered to a localized tumor, producing a higher response rate than intravenous drug administration. The therapeutic index may be further improved by the 'first pass' effect, i.e. extraction of a significant fraction of the administered drug by the tissue fed by the artery. Thus, less drug is available to produce systemic toxicity. The theoretical basis and mathematical principles governing these potential advantages of intraarterial infusions have been outlined by Collins [3], Chen [5] and Eckman [6]. This differential in regional versus systemic concentration is mainly operative during the infusion. Both therapeutic and toxic effects depend on the neoplasm, blood supply and duration of drug levels in tumor and normal tissue drug concentrations [7]. Systemic toxicity depends upon transport rate to the venous circulation, drug excretion and drug metabolism.

Drug levels – concentration gradients in infusional chemotherapy

Chen and Gross described a linear pharmacokinetic model to study drug characteristics after IA and IV infusions predicting the increase in local drug concentration. Tumor drug levels depend upon blood flow rate through the artery and the rate of drug excretion, whereas the systemic drug availability is dependent upon the ability of drug to escape from the infused region. For example, Ensminger et al. demonstrated that the hepatic extraction of a hepatic artery infusion [8] of fluorodeoxyuridine (FUDR) and 5-fluorouracil (5-FU) was on the order of 94–99%, and 19–51% respectively after a single pass through the liver. During hepatic artery infusion, the systemic levels of FUDR and 5-FU were 25 and 60% of corresponding systemic concentrations during peripheral venous infusion. Similar information is available for other drugs and other sites of infusion.

In addition to evaluating the pharmacokinetics in determining the appropriateness of a drug for IA chemotherapy, other factors to be weighed are

Table 1. Criteria for optimal intraarterial chemotherapy.

1. Drug should reach entire tumor bearing area
2. Appropriate drug pharmacokinetics, i.e. steep dose response curve and slow transfer to systemic circulation coupled with rapid systemic excretion
3. Safe, reliable drug delivery system

dose response, schedule, technical adequacy of intraarterial infusion, drug delivery systems and complications. A brief review of major tumor sites treated with infusional chemotherapy will highlight some of these aspects. This area can best be addressed by separating the discussion into hepatic artery infusions versus other arterial infusions of other regions, mainly for treatment of head and neck tumors, extremity tumors (sarcomas and melanomas), and pelvic tumors.

Head and neck cancer and infusional therapy

Head and neck neoplasms generally remain localized or metastasize to regional lymph nodes. The arteries feeding these tumors are readily accessible for selective catheterization. Both characteristics are theoretically ideal for intraarterial treatment of head and neck cancer by infusion chemotherapy. Intravenous single agents methotrexate and cisplatin have achieved response rates of 42 and 26% respectively. Response rates as high as 53 and 60%, respectively, have been reported for intraarterial infusions of these drugs achieved with less systemic toxicity [9, 10]. Response rates ranging from 25 to 80% have been reported for bleomycin, vincristine, and 5-fluorouracil used intraarterially for head and neck malignancies. When choosing intraarterial therapy, the physician must also consider catheter related complications (infection, thrombosis, and bleeding) and the need for hospitalization for both catheter placement and frequently for the infusion itself. Many of these problems have been overcome by use of implantable pumps. Considerable further work must be done before intraarterial infusion becomes a standard therapy for head and neck cancer.

Extremity melanomas and perfusion/infusion therapy

The same rationale discussed previously is applied to using infusional therapy for extremity melanoma [11]. Krementz et al. [12] reported on their large experience with regional perfusion in addition to standard therapy between 1957–1979 in patients with invasive melanoma. Ten-year survival rates were 78% for localized primary disease, 61% for recurrent extremity disease within 3 cm of primary, 28% for skin, soft tissue and nodal disease, and 8% for patients with systemic metastasis. The authors speculate that long term survivors in some of these groups may have been 'cured' with the use of regional drug therapy.

Golomb also reported a better survival in stage III patients treated with surgery with or without perfusion (77% vs. 36%). Stage I patients had no survival benefit, although there was a suggestion of decrease in local recurrences [13]. Complications of limb perfusion in addition to those expected from systemic drug effects include local infection, 'tissue injury', limb edema, vascular damage and neurotoxicity. Regional infusional chemotherapy for limb melanoma should not be considered standard therapy.

Infusional therapy for extremity sarcomas

Sarcomas localized to extremities or pelvis are treatable by intraarterial infusion. Chemotherapy in this setting is generally used in borderline resectable lesions to improve surgical results. The goal is to improve local control, decrease the theoretical risk of metastases during surgery and prolong disease-free survival. Drugs are usually infused pre-operatively thereby identifying effective chemotherapy by measuring gross response as well as degrees of tumor necrosis pathologically [14]. Eilber et al. [15] used intraarterial doxorubicin plus radiation therapy in patients with osteosarcomas. Over 80% of resected specimens showed tumor cell necrosis with more than half showing 90–100% destruction of tumor. Benjamin et al. [16] treated 21 patients with osteosarcoma with pre-op intraarterial cisplatin and systemic doxorubicin followed by resection. In resected specimens, six patients had 100% tumor necrosis and ten patients had greater than 40% tumor necrosis, yielding a total response rate of 76%. Other drugs and schedules are currently being investigated in sarcomas. CT scans, angiography and degree of tumor necrosis are used to assess response with degree of tumor necrosis reported to be the most important predictor of disease-free survival. While this approach seems to have promise, comparative randomized trials are underway at the UCLA to assess superiority to conventionally delivered therapy.

Pelvic tumors and infusional therapy

Intraarterial chemotherapy, usually via the hypogastric arteries for a diverse group of pelvic malignancies has resulted in substantial tumor regression as well as good pain palliation in individual cases. Lathrop reported relief of pain in 74% of patients with a variety of pelvic malignancies treated with intraarterial nitrogen mustard [17]. Response rates of 50% or greater have been reported for various GU tumors treated with intraarterial chemotherapy using 5-fluorouracil, doxorubicin, mitomycin-C and cisplatin [18, 19]. Locally advanced rectal cancer, a relatively common problem, has been treated with intraarterial 5-fluorouracil by Hafstrom whom reported relief of pain in 66% [20]. With the large number of patients with unresectable pelvic malignancies and the limitations of radiation and systemic chemotherapy, infusional therapy appears to be an alternative that deserves further evaluation.

Hepatic artery infusion therapy for colorectal cancer metastatic to the liver

Colorectal cancer is the third most common non-cutaneous malignancy in the United States. The liver is a frequent site of metastasis and may be the only site of evident tumor. Liver metastases are associated with a very poor prognosis and are also a major source of morbidity in this group of patients. Therapeutic options in this setting including resection, intravenous chemotherapy, radiation and embolization have been beneficial only in the minority of patients. Regional chemotherapy via the hepatic artery has many appealing theoretical advantages and has been under study since the 1960s [21].

Rationale for hepatic artery infusion therapy

The potential usefulness of hepatic artery infusion therapy is based upon the differential blood supply in the liver between metastatic tumor nodules (which derive most of their blood supply from the hepatic artery) and the liver parenchyma predominantly supplied by the portal circulation. Thus, drug infused through the hepatic artery allows a higher drug concentration to tumor capillaries than to hepatocytes [22]. A second factor enhancing the attractiveness of hepatic artery infusions for certain drugs is the 'first pass phenomenon'. When a drug has a high percent hepatic extraction, a significant fraction is removed during the drug's first pass through the liver resulting in lower systemic levels and less toxicity. FUDR, for example has a 94% extraction during its first pass [23]. Schedule for certain drugs is also critical. Because the fluoropyrimidines are cell cycle active, for example, continuous infusion of these agents should result in a greater cell kill.

Several large studies using external pumps have been published [24–26]. In general, reported response rates of liver metastases are higher than with the use of systemic drugs; however, these studies are flawed due to poor definition of extent of disease and response criteria. Technical complications associated with using external pumps and catheters have limited acceptance of this mode of intraarterial therapy.

Implantable systems

Recently, totally implantable drug infusion pumps have been developed,

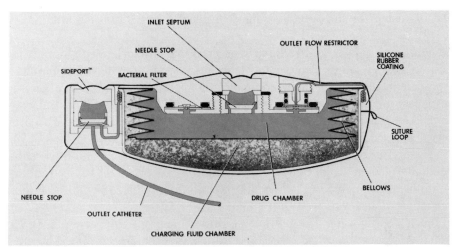

Figure 2. Schematic model of infusaid (R) implantable pump (Infusaid Corp., Norwood, Massachusetts), and example of a totally implantable pump drug delivery system.

making long-term arterial infusion therapy technically more feasible and aesthetically more acceptable [27]. An example of a totally implantable drug infusion pump, the Infusaid (R) pump (Figure 2) was developed in the early 70s to deliver heparin to patients with thromboembolic disease. It has subsequently become approved for infusion of floxuridine into the hepatic artery. The pump system is comprised of a titanium cylinder separated into two chambers by metal bellows. One chamber, permanently sealed between the bellows and outside wall of the cylinder, contains a two phase (gas-liquid) charging fluid. The other chamber is a drug reservoir that can be filled via a subcutaneously positioned septum. With the drug reservoir filled, the charging fluid is compressed into a liquid state. As it is warmed by the patient's body temperature, it becomes a vapor exerting a pressure on the drug filled reservoir, forcing the drug out into the catheter at a constant flow rate. Pumps also can contain a sideport to administer bolus injections of drugs or radionuclides to assess drug flow to a given region. A double catheter system is also available. The silicon catheters may be placed into the artery feeding the tumor. The pump itself is implanted in a subcutaneous pocket. The surgical technique for implanting this pump has been well described [27]. Advantages to an implantable system include: (1) lower rate of infection, thrombosis and catheter malfunction; (2) therapy can be delivered as an outpatient after initial implantation; (3) little necessary maintenance; (4) high patient acceptance and; (5) long pump life. The major disadvantages include; (1) initial cost of implantation ($ 3000–$ 6000 per pump); (2) inability to reuse the pump for other patients; (3) flow rate which varies with barometric and temperature changes; and (4) a limited reservoir volume.

Results using the implantable pumps in hepatic artery infusion studies

Several randomized studies have suggested that intraarterial therapy using an implantable pump results in a higher response rate of hepatic metastases from colorectal cancer than conventional therapy. However, the gain in response rate of intrahepatic metastasis appeared to be offset by extrahepatic disease progression. The survival was similar in both groups. The drug regimens used are shown in Table 2. Niederhuber et al. [28] reported objective responses of 83% as measured by CEA, physical exams and liver scans. Median survival from pump implantation is reported to be 18 months. Complications included gastritis, ulcers, and drug-induced hepatitis. Pump-related complications were infrequent.

Balch [29] reported a response rate of 88% (using CEA decrements). No major complications were reported. Death was secondary to tumor progression extrahepatically in most patients.

Kemeny et al. [30] have reported a response rate of 39% for hepatic artery infusion but emphasized toxicity. Gastritis and hepatitis often necessitated discontinued treatment. The influence of performance status and extent of liver disease were emphasized as significant prognostic indicators of survival. This group recently updated their randomized trial of intrahepatic versus systemic infusion of flurodeoxyuridine (FUDR) in patients with liver metastases from colorectal cancer [31]. The two groups were well matched. At the time of this report, median survival is similar, 15 months in both groups and although the interim response rate is higher in the hepatic group, survival is identical.

Table 2. Results of intraarterial chemotherapy using implantable pump in patients with hepatic metastases from colorectal cancer.

	Regimen	Response rate	Median survival from pump implantation
Niederhuber et al. [31]	FUDR 0.3 mg/kg × 14 d then NS × 14 d	83%	18 mos.
Kemeny et al. [33]	FUDR 0.3 mg/kg/d × 14 then NS × 14 d	39%	–
Balch et al. [32]	FUDR 0.3 mg/kg × 14 d then NS × 14 d	88%	26 mos.*
Cohen et al. [34]	FUDR 0.3 mg/kg × 14 d	54%	12 mos.

* From diagnosis of metastases.

Cohen et al. [32] reported 45 patients who had undergone pump implants. Of 39 evaluable patients, 54% responded based on physical exam and liver scans.

Drugs other than FUDR are being infused through the hepatic artery. Bertino et al. reported early results with a phase I-II study using sequential dichloromethotrexate and 5-fluorouracil given via the hepatic artery to patients with colon cancer metastatic to liver [33]. Numbers of patients are small, three of four evaluable patients have had disease stabilization with improvement in performance status and additional patients are being accrued to this study.

Comments on hepatic artery infusion therapy

While these data are encouraging, reported response rates vary considerably as does patient selection and response criteria. Toxicity can be substantial (particularly cholangitis) and extrahepatic disease remains a major obstacle. Many questions remain to be answered including optimal drug choice, and duration of therapy. Indications for hepatic arterial chemotherapy, if any, will hopefully be precisely defined by prospective controlled clinical trials currently underway, to assess response, survival, quality of life and long-term toxicities [34].

Third-space chemotherapy: overview

Some tumors characteristically diffusely invade body cavities (third spaces), where they can cause significant morbidity and ultimately mortality. Affected cavities include the peritoneal, pleural, pericardial and cerebrospinal fluid (CSF) space. These spaces are separated from the blood stream by a diffusion barrier resulting in 'pharmacologic sanctuaries'. In the last decade, a formal body of pharmacokinetic theory has been developed pertaining to administration of drug into the CSF space [35, 36], and the peritoneal cavity [37, 38]. These principles can generally be applied to the pleural and pericardial space as well [39]. Factors influencing the success of this form of therapy include drug distribution within the cavity, tumor penetration, disease volume, sensitivity of the tumor to available agents and access to the cavities [40]. Compared to intraarterial delivery, intracavitary routes have more favorable regional exchange rates (i.e. less systemic drug for a given intracavitary concentration), but they also have a different pattern of drug distribution to local tissues [41]. All tissues supplied by the artery infused are exposed to an increased drug concentration whereas only tissues that contact third space fluid are exposed to the full increase in drug concentration produced by the intracavitary route. This concentration differential decreases quickly only a few millimeters from the tissue surface.

Intraperitoneal (IP) therapy – general principles of third space chemotherapy

Much of the available data on intraperitoneal chemotherapy comes from IP treatment of ovarian cancer. Many ovarian cancer patients present with or develop widespread seeding of the peritoneal surfaces resulting in major morbidity. Although ovarian cancer is quite sensitive to a variety of drugs, cure may be prevented because the peritoneum becomes a pharmacologic 'sanctuary site'. While IP chemotherapy in ovarian cancer may be used to palliate ascites, current studies are attempting to define whether it has a role in the overall management of earlier stages of ovarian cancer. Questions similar to those being studied in intraarterial therapy are also relevant here: (1) Does IP therapy result in a significant response rate? (2) What drug(s) should be used? (3) To which diseases and stages should it be applied? (4) What is the technically optimal method to deliver IP drugs? These questions are currently under study. Direct drug instillation into the peritoneal cavity results in higher local drug concentrations which may improve the therapeutic index. The resulting concentration gradient is proportional to the ratio of total-body clearance to peritoneal clearance [37]. Peritoneal clearance of most drugs correlates inversely with its molecular weight, (higher molecular weights result in slower absorption). Actual clearances have been calculated for a number of drugs. Resulting concentration differentials range from 10 to 2000 (Table 3). There may also be a range for an individual drug depending on peritoneal permeability, systemic clearances, initial concentration, or other factors. Thus, the ideal drug for intraperitoneal use would have a large concentration gradient advantage, a steep dose response curve for the tumor being treated, and little local toxicity. A perfect agent does not exist but several agents are under active investigation.

Table 3. Pharmacologic advantage for various drugs given intraperitoneally, i.e. peak peritoneal drug concentration over systemic IV drug concentration.

Drug	Measured concentration differentials	Ref.
5-Fluorouracil	550–7852	53
Doxorubicin	474	46
Cisplatin	21	44
Methotrexate	7–303	40

Specific drugs used intraperitoneally

Cisplatin

Cisplatin (cis-diamino-dichloro-platinum II) is a small molecule that leaves the peritoneal cavity quickly and is relatively slowly cleared, thus yielding a relatively small concentration advantage. In an attempt to improve upon the therapeutic index, Howell et al. used higher doses of cisplatin intraperitoneally with peripherally infused thiosulfate to inactivate platinum systemically [42]. However, this study was unable to show a steep dose response curve in patients with ovarian cancer. On the other hand, Corden reported evidence of a dose response in ovarian cancer; an increased response rate in patients was obtained with the doubling of the dose of cisplatin [43].

In contrast to most other agents, intraperitoneal cisplatin has not been associated with chemical peritonitis. The absence of local toxicity and the demonstration of activity in phase II trials, makes cisplatin an attractive drug for further study of intraperitoneal chemotherapy in patients with ovarian cancer.

Doxorubicin

Although an active drug, doxorubicin is a vesicant. Its dose-limiting toxicity in a phase I trial at NCI was chemical peritonitis. However, a large concentration gradient can be obtained and several responses were observed in a group with heavily pretreated ovarian cancer [44]. Further clinical evaluation is warranted.

5-Fluorouracil

5-FU has been used successfully given intraperitoneally to control ascites since 1965 [45]. About 70% of IP 5-FU subsequently appears in the portal vein. This may be theoretically advantageous for the adjuvant treatment of high risk colon cancer patients, treating peritoneal seeding and microscopic liver metastases [46]. Sugarbaker et al., at NCI, reported recently on a prospective randomized trial of intravenous versus intraperitoneal 5-fluorouracil in patients with advanced colon or rectal cancer [47]. A higher dose of 5-fluorouracil was achieved with the intraperitoneal route without an increase in adverse side effects. In this study, the natural history of surgically treated disease was changed by reducing the incidence of peritoneal carcinomatosis in those patients treated with intraperitoneal 5-fluorouracil. However, the time to relapse and survival was not greater than for those receiving intravenous 5-fluorouracil. Sigurdson et al. report demonstrating FUDR uptake by tumor following portal vein infusion is negligible compared to hepatic artery infusion [48]. This may help explain why there was no difference in liver as a site of failure in Sugarbaker's study. It is recommended that IP 5-fluorouracil continue to be used investigationally or as one part of a multimodality treatment protocol for colorectal cancer.

Methotrexate

Theoretical advantages to regional methotrexate therapy have been elegantly described. However, clinical results are conflicting. Methotrexate can also cause significant chemical peritonitis [39, 40]. However, Howell et al. [39] reported dramatic responses to intracavitary methotrexate including a case of lung cancer involving the pleural space.

Other drugs

Intraperitoneal melphalan, bleomycin and cytosine arabinoside have been studied [50, 51]. Other drugs and combinations of drugs are currently undergoing investigation.

Access to the peritoneal cavity

Repeated percutaneous paracentesis can be associated with bowel perforation, peritonitis, and occasional bleeding. The Tenckoff catheter, initially developed for intraperitoneal dialysis, has been used for drug delivery but is not ideal because of the high rate of peritonitis, the need for frequent biweekly flushing, and poor patient acceptance (due to the external catheter there is a need for sterile technique and there are shower and swimming limitations). Semipermanent indwelling catheters placed in the peritoneal cavity can be connected to a subcutaneous access device, e.g. a Port-A-Cath (R) (Pharmacia N.J.) [52]. These systems are accessed transcutaneously and require little maintenance. While the risk for infection appears to be decreased in comparison to Tenckoff catheters, indwelling catheters frequently develop a one way valve malfunction (i.e., drugs can be delivered but specimens cannot be obtained from the peritoneal catheter). Because of lumen size, rates of flow may be quite slow. Unlike the Tenckoff catheter which may be easily removed percutaneously, subcutaneous catheters require surgical removal. Modifications of currently available catheter systems may even allow safer more efficient delivery.

Drug distribution

The optimal distribution of drug throughout the peritoneal cavity is frequently impossible because of adhesions or tumor masses. Instillation of a radionuclide followed by imaging or Hypaque followed by CT scan have both been used to assess drug distribution intraperitoneally, and at times have permitted visualization of tumor nodules [53]. Relatively large fluid volumes have been shown to assure optimal drug distribution.

IP therapy has been infused rapidly, as a continuous infusion [54] or via exchange dialysis. The choice depends on the drug, patient convenience, the catheter system used and available pumps.

Drug levels

The drug concentration can be adjusted to produce no systemic effects or a toxicity comparable to that achieved with a standard IV dose or even to produce maximally tolerated blood levels. In some cases IP drug levels of 10- to 2000-fold higher than IV levels can be achieved. The IP dose could be escalated to dose-limiting toxicity, or IP and IV drug could be simultaneously administered. Attaining high IP and systemic drug levels theoretically may overcome drug diffusion limitations and treat extra-regional disease simultaneously. Overall responses have been reported with this type of therapy in heavily pretreated ovarian cancer patients, thus consideration should be given to evaluating IP therapy in less heavily treated patients (Table 4).

Table 4. Responses reported for IP therapy in the treatment of previously treated ovarian cancer.

	Drug	Responses
Howell et al. [44]	cisplatin	1/7
Ozals et al. [46]	doxorubicin	3/10
Howell et al. [40]	methotrexate	2/2
Gyves et al. [52]	5-fluorouracil	1/5

Concluding remarks on intraperitoneal chemotherapy

While malignant ascites can be controlled in many cases, the ultimate value of IP drug therapy remains to be defined. Other indications for IP therapy may eventually include adjuvant therapy for early ovarian cancer or colon cancer, or IP delivery after surgical debulking of more advanced ovarian cancer or as an alternative to hepatic artery infusion for liver metastases. Intraperitoneal therapy may also be appropriate to treat bulk disease if therapeutic blood levels are also attained [40]. The major limitation of IP therapy is the need for systemic therapy if: (1) tumor has seeded beyond the peritoneum and (2) tumor has grown to more than a few millimeters in size because the drug must diffuse into the tumor mass [55]. Technical improvements may enhance the study of IP drug delivery. Pharmacology and toxicology of IP drug delivery are developing. New drugs and drug analogues are being tested in phase I trials. Well designed clinical trials are now needed to determine the value of this approach.

Other third spaces

Intrathecal therapy has been thoroughly established both in the adjuvant setting in acute lymphoblastic leukemia and in established meningeal leukemia [56] or in the palliative treatment of carcinomatous meningitis. Pleural and pericardial spaces are other areas where intracavitary instillation of drug holds promise [39, 57, 58]. Treatment has been mainly aimed at palliation, especially in the control of symptomatic effusions. Intracavitary therapy may play a larger role in these areas as repeated access to these cavities becomes technically feasible.

Conclusion

Regional drug delivery is one of several approaches toward improved anticancer chemotherapy based on the laboratory observation of a linear-log dose response curve i.e. doubling the dose of a given agent results in up to 10-fold higher cell kill. A higher drug concentration delivered regionally may overcome drug resistance locally and yet reduce systemic toxicity. The pharmacologic basis for regional chemotherapy has been and continues to be developed.

Major problems remain: technical difficulties, extra-regional tumor growth, and toxicities. However, the established role of intrathecal therapy and the positive initial experience with intraperitoneal therapy in ovarian cancer suggest a role for regional infusion in the future.

Certain available data suggests that while hepatic artery infusion may result in an enhanced response rate, because of extra regional tumor growth, this type of 'high tech' treatment has not resulted in prolonged survival. Stablein [59] however has observed that common end points in many studies are to 'cure' or extend survival. However, in diseases where the goal of cure is still ellusive, perhaps objectives should be more limited, such as the control of ascites or preservation of hepatic function. Treatment with these less ambitious goals can provide useful information. Thus, while cure or even prolonged survival may be unrealistic goals for the initial evaluation of new treatment methods, palliation of symptoms and maintenance or improvement of the quality of life should not be overlooked as valid study and therapeutic end points.

References

1. Frei E, Canellos GP. 1980. Dose: A critical factor in cancer chemotherapy. Am J Med 69:585–594.
2. Ensminger WD, Gyves JW. 1984. Regional cancer chemotherapy. Cancer Treat Rep 68:101–115.
3. Collins JM. 1984. Pharmacologic rationale for regional drug delivery. J Clin Oncol 2:498–504.
4. Klopp CT, Alford TC, Bateman et al. 1950. Fractionated intra-arterial cancer chemotherapy with methyl histamine hydrochloride. Preliminary Report. Ann Surg 132:811–832.
5. Chen HG, Gross JF. 1980. Intraarterial infusion of anticancer drugs: Theoretic aspects of drug delivery and review of responses. Cancer Treat Rep 64:31–40.
6. Eckman WW, Patlak CS, Fenstermacher JD. 1974. A critical evaluation of principles governing the advantages of intraarterial infusions. J Pharmakokinet Biopharm 2:257–285.
7. Wallace, Sidney et al. 1984. Percutaneous transcatheter infusion and infarction in the treatment of human cancer: Part 1. Curr Probl Cancer pp 1–66, Dec.
8. Ensminger WD, Rosowsky A, Raso V et al. 1978. A clinical pharmacologic evaluation of hepatic arterial infusions of 5-Fluoro-2-deoxyuridine and 5-fluorouracil. Cancer Res 38:3784–3792.
9. Freckman HA. 1972. Results in 169 patients with cancer of the head and neck treated by intra-arterial infusion therapy. Am J Surg 124:501–509.
10. Baker SR, Wheeler R. 1982. Long term intraarterial chemotherapy infusion of head and neck cancer patients. J Surg Oncol 21:125–131.
11. Sutherland CM, Krementz ET. 1982. The role in limb perfusion in the management of malignant melanoma. Post graduate course. Surg Oncol Today pp 119–121.
12. Krementz ET, Carter RD, Sutherland EM et al. 1979. The use of chemotherapy in the management of malignant melanoma. World J Surg 3:289–304.
13. Golomb FM. 1976. Perfusion in cancer of the skin. In: Biology, diagnosis, management, Vol. II. Andrade R, Gumport SL, Popkin GL, Rees TD (eds). Philadelphia, W.B. Saunders CO., p 1623.
14. Rosen G, Marcove RC, Huvos AG et al. 1983. Primary osteogenic sarcoma: eight year experience with adjuvant chemotherapy. J Cancer Res Clin Oncol 106 (Suppl):55–67.
15. Eilber FR, Grant T, Morton DL. 1978. Adjuvant therapy for osteosarcoma: Pre-operative treatment. Cancer Treat Rep 62:213–216.

72

16. Benjamin RS, Chuang VP, Wallace S, Murray J et al. 1982. Pre-operative chemotherapy for osteosarcoma. Proc ASCO 23:174 (C-675).
17. Lathrop JC, Frates RC. 1980. Arterial infusion of nitrogen mustard in the treatment of intractable pelvic pain of malignant origin. Cancer (Feb) 45:432–438.
18. Wallace S, Chuang VP, Samuels M, Johnson D. 1982. Transcatheter intraarterial infusion of chemotherapy in advanced bladder cancer. Cancer (Feb 15) 40(4):640–645.
19. Logothetis CT, Samuels ML, Wallard S, Chuang V et al. 1982. Management of pelvic complications of malignant urothelial tumors with combined intraarterial and intravenous chemotherapy. Cancer Treat Rep 66:1501–1507.
20. Hafstrom L, Johnson PE, Landberg T et al. 1979. Intraarterial infusion of chemotherapy (5-FU) in patients with inextirpable or locally recurrent rectal cancer. Am J Surg (June) pp 757–762.
21. Sullivan RD, Norcross JW, Watkins E Jr. 1964. Chemotherapy of metastatic liver cancer by prolonged hepatic artery infusion. N Engl J Med 270:321–327.
22. Bierman HR, Poyron RL, Kelley KH et al. 1951. Studies on the blood supplies of tumors in man. Vascular patterns of the liver by hepatic arteriography in vivo. J Natl Cancer Inst 12:107–181.
23. Ensminger WD, Rosowsky A, Raso V et al. 1978. A Clinical pharmacological evaluation of hepatic arterial infusions of 5-fluoro-2'-deoxyuridine and 5-fluorouracil. Cancer Res 38:3784–3792.
24. Watkins E, Khazer AM, Nahra KS. 1970. Surgical basis for arterial infusion chemotherapy of disseminated carcinoma of the liver. Surg Gynecol Obstet 120:581–605.
25. Cady B, Oberfield RA. 1974. Regional infusion chemotherapy of hepatic metastases from carcinoma of the colon. Am J Surg 127:220–227.
26. Reed ML, Vaitkevicias VK, Al-Sarraf M et al. 1981. The practicality of chronic hepatic artery infusion therapy of primary and metastatic hepatic malignancies. Cancer 47:402–409.
27. Ensminger W, Niederhuber J, Dakhil S et al. 1981. Totally implanted drug delivery system for hepatic artery chemotherapy. Cancer Treat Rep 65:393–400.
28. Niederhuben, JE, Ensminger W, Gyves J. 1984. Regional chemotherapy of colorectal cancer metastatic to liver Cancer 53:1336–1345.
29. Balch CM, Urest MM, Soong S et al. 1983. A prospective phase II clinical trial of continuous FUDR regional chemotherapy for colorectal metastases to the liver using a totally implantable drug infusion pump. Am Surg 198:567–573.
30. Kemeny N, Daly JM, Oderman P et al. 1983. Hepatic infusion chemotherapy for metastatic colorectal carcinoma, results and complications. Proc ASCO 2:123 (C-482).
31. Kemeny N, Reichman B, Oderman J et al. 1986. Update of randomized study of intrahepatic (H) vs systemic (S) infusion of flurodeoxyuridine (FUDR) in patients with liver metastases from colorectal carcinoma (CRC). Proc Asco 5:89 (C-345).
32. Cohen Am, Kaufman SD, Wood WC et al. 1983. Regional hepatic chemotherapy using an implantable drug infusin pump. Am J Surg 145:529–533.
33. Bertino JR, Lacy J et al. 1986. A phase I-II trial of intrahepatic (IH) sequential dichloromethotrexate (DCM) and 5-fluorouracil (5-FU) chemotherapy for colon cancer metastatic to liver. Proc ASCO 5:94 (C-365).
34. Stagg RJ, Lewis BJ, Friedman MA, Ignoffo RJ, Hohn DC. 1984. Hepatic arterial chemotherapy for colorectal cancer metastatic to the liver. Review Ann Intern Med 100:736–743.
35. Shapiro WR, Young DF, Mehta BM. 1975. Methotrexate: distribution in cerebrospinal fluid after intravenous, ventricular and lumbar injections. N Engl J Med 293:101–166.
36. Blasberg R, Patlak C, Fenstermacher J et al. 1975. Intrathecal chemotherapy: Brain tissue profiles after ventriculo-cisternal perfusion. Perfusion J Pharmacol Exp Ther 195:73–83.

37. Dedrick RL, Myers CE, Bungay PM et al. 1978. Pharmacokinetic rational for peritoneal drug administration in the treatment of ovarian cancer. Cancer Treat Rep 62:1-11.
38. Myers C, Collins J. 1983. Pharmacology of intraperitoneal chemotherapy. Cancer Invest 1:395-407.
39. Howell S, Chu B, Wung W et al. 1981. Long duration intracavitary infusion of Methotrexate with systemic Leucovorin protection in patients with malignant effusions. J Clin Invest 67:1161-1170.
40. Myers C. 1984. The use of intraperitoneal chemotherapy in the treatment of ovarian cancer. Sem Oncol 11:275-284.
41. Collins JM. 1984. Pharmacologic rationale for regional drug delivery. J Clin Oncol 2:498-504.
42. Howell SB, Pfeifle CE, Wung WE, Olshen RA. 1983. Intraperitoneal Cis-diaminedichloroplatinum with systemic thiosulfate protection. Cancer Res 43:1476-1531.
43. Corden BJ, Hill JB, Collins J, Ozols RF. 1983. High dose Cis-Platinum in hypertonic saline absence of nephrotoxicity and pharmacokinetic of 40 mg/m^2 × 5 schedule of administration. Proc ASCO 2:34 (C-132).
44. Ozols RF, Young RC, Speyer JL, Sugarbaker PH, Greene R, Jenkins J, Myers CE. 1982. Phase I and pharmacologic studies of Adriamycin intraperitoneally in patients with ovarian cancer. Cancer Res. 42:4265-4269.
45. Suhrland LG, Weisberger AS. 1965. Intracavitary 5-fluorouracil in malignant effusions. Arch. Intern. Med. 116:431-433.
46. Speyer JL, Sugarbaker PH, Collins JM et al. 1985. Portal levels and hepatic clearance of 5-fluorouracil after intraperitoneal administration in humans. Cancer Res 41:1916-1922.
47. Sugarbaker PH, Gianola FJ, Speyer JL et al. 1985. Prospective randomized trial of intravenous vs intraperitoneal 5-fluorouracil in patients with advanced primary colon or rectal cancer. Surgery 98:414-421.
48. Sigurdson ER, Ridge JA, Kemeny N, Daly JM. 1986. Comparison of drug uptake of colorectal hepatic metastases after hepatic artery and portal vein infusion. Proc ASCO 5:266 (C-1039).
49. Jones RB, Collins JM, Myers CC et al. 1981. High volume intraperitoneal chemotherapy with Methotrexate in patients with cancer. Cancer Res 41:55-59.
50. Alberts DS, Chen HSG, Chang SY, Peng YM. 1980. The disposition of intraperitoneal Bleomycin, Melphalan, and Vinblastine in cancer. Recent results. Cancer Res 74:293-299.
51. Mackman M, Cleary S, Lucas W, Howell S. 1985. Intraperitoneal chemotherapy with high dose Cis-Platinum and Cytosine Arabinoside for refractory ovarian carcinoma and other malignancies principally involving the peritoneal cavity. J Clin Oncol 3:925-931.
52. Pfeifle CE, Howell SB, Markman M et al. 1984. Totally implantable system for peritoneal access. J Clin Oncol 2:1277-1280.
53. Dunnick N, Jones R, Doppman J et al. 1979. Intraperitoneal contrast infusion for assessment of intraperitoneal fluid dynamics. AJR 133:221-223.
54. Gyves J, Ensminger W, Stetson P et al. 1984. Constant intraperitoneal 5-fluorouracil infusion through a totally imlanted system. Clin Pharmacol Ther 35:83-89.
55. Myers C. 1985. The use of intraperitoneal chemotherapy. In: Important Advances in Oncology (Devita V, Hellman S, Rosenberg S, eds). Lippincott Co, Philadelphia, pp 218-225.
56. Bleyer WA, Poplack DG. 1985. Prophylaxis and treatment of leukemia in the central nervous system and other sactuaries. Oncol 12:131-148 (June).
57. Paladine W et al. 1976. Intracavitary bleomycin in the management of malignant effusions. Cancer 38:1903-1908.
58. Theologides A. 1978. Neoplastic cardiac tamponade. Sem Oncol 5:181-192.
59. Stablein Donald. 1985. Statistical aspects of intraperitoneal chemotherapy studies. Sem Oncol XII, 3:121-123 (Sept).

6. Use of hyperthermia for treatment of malignant disease; biologic rationale, techniques, clinical results

RONALD S. SCOTT

Introduction

Interest in the use of hyperthermia in the treatment of malignant disease is first recorded in the German literature in the middle of the late 19th century [1, 2]. These investigators noticed the serendipitous regression of tumors following infections such as erysipilas. Investigators during the next several decades continued this interest both by making note of tumor response secondary to high fevers such as those accompanying certain infections as well as by the actual induction of such infections, for instance plasmodial infections, which led to an actual clinical trial of hyperthermia with Warren's induction of fever by deliberate infection in 1935 [3]. Attempts to selectively heat tumors in patients were hampered by technological constraints. The most straightforward techniques involved placing patients in a heated environment (e.g., saunas or hot water baths), but these resulted in excessive skin temperatures before core temperatures or tumor temperatures reached therapeutic levels. The technologic development which had the greatest impact on patient hyperthermia was electronic or radiofrequency heating. These techniques involve a high degree of electronic sophistication and therefore have been pioneered by physicians who commonly use such modalities in their approach to patients, namely radiologists or radiation oncologists. While the initial emphasis on the use of heat in the treatment of malignant disease addressed the response of the tumor to the effect of heat alone, it was only natural that radiation oncologists should explore the possible synergy between electronically generated hyperthermia treatments and more established cytotoxic effects of ionizing radiation commonly used in their speciality. As such synergy has been demonstrated in cell culture, animal models, and most recently, controlled patient trials, explorations of synergy between hyperthermia and cytotoxic chemotherapeutic agents are now being vigorously undertaken. Such studies are primarily in the laboratory stage at this time but interest in this mode of therapy is rapidly expanding.

Higby, DJ (ed), Issues in Supportive Care of Cancer Patients. ISBN 0-89838-816-3.
© *1986, Martinus Nijhoff Publishers, Boston. Printed in the Netherlands.*

Hyperthermia in combination with radiation therapy

Several preclinical studies predicted that a synergy between hyperthermia and radiotherapy in the clinical setting would be found [4–11]. Among the areas where this synergy has been especially demonstrated is an enhanced response to heat and radiation on proliferating cells in the S-phase of the cell cycle. Gerwick et al. [4] examined the effect of combined hyperthermia and radiotherapy on synchronous cell cultures *in vitro*. Cell survival curves were generated following radiotherapy in each segment of the cell cycle. For cells in G_1 the cytotoxic effects of each modality were additive, but no synergy was demonstrated. For cells in S-phase, following heat, the radiation survival curve demonstrated a reduced D_0, indicating an enhanced radiosensitivity as a result of hyperthermia. When the effect of hyperthermia on the radiosensitivity of these cells in G_1 and S were compared without hyperthermia, cells in G_1 are more sensitive to radiation than cells in S. However, after hyperthermia treatment, cells in S-phase are more sensitive to radiation than are cells in G, and the primary mechanism of this increased sensitivity is a reduced shoulder on the cell survival curve for S-phase cells. When the shoulder of a radiation cell survival curve is reduced along with a reduced D_0, it is inferred that the cell's capability to repair sublethal damage has been impaired. Ben Hur et al. [5, 6], in fact, had previously suggested a reduction in a cycling cell's capacity to accumulate sub-lethal damage as a potential mechanism of synergy between radiotherapy and hyperthermia.

Dewey et al. [7], Freeman et al. [8] and Dewhirst et al. [9] addressed the possible benefit hyperthermia might have in overcoming the traditional radiotherapeutic dilemma of the relative insensitivity of chronically hypoxic cells to the cytotoxic effects of ionizing radiation. These workers determined that while hypoxic cells per se are not substantially more sensitive to the combination of hyperthermia and radiotherapy, cells maintained at low pH are far more sensitive to the combination than are cells at physiologic pH. A hypoxic sanctuary from ionizing radiation is almost invariably associated with reduced pH rendering this compartment particularly sensitive to the synergistic effects of hyperthermia and radiotherapy. Stewart et al. [10] further demonstrated that tumors made chronically hypoxic and respired to low pH were far more sensitive to the combination of hyperthermia and radiotherapy than to radiotherapy alone.

Sapareto et al. [11], in a study primarily addressing thermal tolerance, noted that at temperatures as low as 41.5 °C cycling cells were arrested in the G_1 phase with no DNA synthesis taking place for more than 20 h, while DNA synthesis would have been expected at 8–10 h without heating. Moreover, there was a redistribution in the cell cycle in favor of cells in the G_2- and M-phase at the expense of cells in the S-phase. The net result of these two events would be to increase the radioresponsiveness of this cell population. Cells in S-phase are generally more resistant to radiotherapy than cells in G_2- and M-phase, and an arrest in G_1-phase reduces the repopulation of the cells' mass, reducing the burden on the cytotoxic technique needed to sterilize the cell mass. For this reason, even mild hyperthermia, as might be obtained in selected, well vascularized regions of a given tumor, can be expected to induce radiosensitization in a cycling cell population.

Tumor studies

Robinson et al. [12] examined the effect of ionizing radiation and heat on both normal skin of mice as well as tumors. They defined the therapeutic enhancement ratio (TER) as the TER for normal tissue which was determined to be unity at a temperature of 40.3 °C and increased to 2.06 at 43 °C. They repeated the study for tumor and showed that at 40.4 °C the TER was again unity, but increased to 4.33 at 43 °C. The slopes of the TER of normal tissue and tumor vs. temperature were both linear. A therapeutic gain factor can be defined as the TER of tumor divided by the TER of normal tissue. According to this group's results, this therapeutic gain factor is unity at 40.3 °C and rises linearly to approximately 2.1 at 43 °C. This very compelling result implies a definite synergy between simultaneously applied hyperthermia and ionizing radiation.

Overgaard [13] made a detailed study of the sequencing of hyperthermia and radiation therapy treatments on experimental tumors. TER, in his study, was determined to be slightly more than unity at 41 °C for 60 min and rose to nearly 5 at 43.5 °C for 60 min. However, he failed to demonstrate a therapeutic gain factor when hyperthermia and radiotherapy were given simultaneously. When the radiotherapy was given after the hyperthermia, there was an increase in the therapeutic gain factor, although the TER for both tumor and normal tissue declined. The therapeutic gain factor was determined to attain a maximum value of 1.5 when a 4-h period separated heat and radiotherapy. A definite improvement in the therapeutic gain factor was demonstrated when as little as one hour separated the application of the two modalities.

Emami et al. [14, 15] showed that dilatation and congestion of the microvasculature could be expected shortly after an exposure of 40.5 °C for 40 min. Definite dilatation and congestion resulted from treatment at 43.5 °C for 40 min, this change progressing to some evidence of vascular rupture. When 44.5 °C was applied for 40 min, definite vascular rupture was determined and frank coagulation necrosis was demonstrated. Eddy et al. [16, 17] examined the effect of hyperthermia on tumor microvasculature *in vitro/in situ* and essentially confirmed the results of Enami et al., whose study had required histologic sectioning of the heated tumor. Eddy demonstrated that 45 °C for 30 min produced immediate changes in the microvasculature resulting in non-functional vessels at 24 h and typical coagulation necrosis at 48 h. Song et al. [18], using radiolabeled microspheres and red blood cells, also demonstrated major damage to the microvasculature for tumors heated in the 43–45 °C range. All of these studies suggest that in addition to the synergy between hyperthermia and radiotherapy at the cellular level, there are also direct tumorocidal effects of hyperthermia resulting from vascular damage in areas of the tumor where perfusion is limited or marginal, the very sites which are sanctuaries from the cytotoxic effects of ionizing radiation.

Several workers [19–23] have demonstrated and attempted to elucidate thermal tolerance. Cells which have been heated become resistant to further heat treatments given shortly after the initial treatment. This resistance is most pronounced approximately 5 h after the treatment and progressively decays over a period of several days. Various investigators have determined this decay to be essentially complete, cells being no longer thermally tolerant, at periods varying between 72 and 120 h. Thermal tolerance has been established to be a result of heat shock proteins synthesized by the cell in response to the thermal shock. The degradation of these proteins probably occurs over the time period for which thermal tolerance has been demonstrated. The clinical implication of this effect is that rapid fractionation of heat treatments is likely to be counterproductive in the treatment of malignant tumors.

Hyperthermia and chemotherapy

While the combination of hyperthermia and chemotherapy is a logical extension of its use with radiotherapy, knowledge of the interaction is far less well developed. Detailed experimental data is currently only available *in vitro*. For the purposes of this description, cytotoxic chemotherapeutic agents are divided into three categories. First, there are those which increase in cytoxicity linearly with increasing temperature; these include the alkylating agents, cisplatin and mitomycin-C. Second, there is a class of agents whose cytotoxicity is enhanced only above a threshold temperature, typically 41 to 42 °C. These drugs include doxorubicin, bleomycin, and actinomycin-D. Third, there are drugs which are not commonly associated with cytotoxicity at 37 °C, but become cytotoxic at temperature higher than 41 to 42 °C. The prototype drug in this category is the anti-fungal agent amphotericin-B. Commonly used chemotherapeutic agents which do not show increased cytotoxicity with increasing temperature include 5-fluorouracil and the various Vinca alkaloids.

The interactions between hyperthermia and chemotherapeutic agents is further complicated by the way in which these agents interact. Insofar as a cytotoxic drug must be present in the intracellular compartment to act, membrane permeability will affect drug activity. Hyperthermia is known to exert a substantial effect on the cell membrane. For this reason, the sequencing of hyperthermia and various cytotoxic agents could be critical in any synergy which might be produced. A group of experiments has been performed and reported which illustrate the complexity of the problem of demonstrating synergy between hyperthermia and chemotherapy as well as designing a rational protocol for their use. Hahn et al. [24] showed that when treating Chinese hamster ovary cells, simultaneous exposure to heat and doxorubicin produced synergism; however, if the cells were exposed to heat prior to doxorubicin administration, the cytotoxic effect of the anthrocycline is reduced. If treatment with hyperthermia increases cell membrane permeability one would expect that either simultaneous administration of hyperthermia and doxorubicin or doxorubicin following hyperthermia would demonstrate synergism whereas doxorubicin administration preceding hyperthermia would be unlikely to demonstrate such a synergism. The observation that doxorubicin administration following hyperthermic treatment resulted in a lower cytotoxic effect from doxorubicin was originally poorly explained. However, current knowledge of heat shock proteins provides an explanation for this effect. Cells treated with hyperthermia develop thermal tolerance as a result of the elucidation of heat-shock proteins which begins during and in the immediate post-treatment period. Heat-shock proteins act in many ways to stabilize the cell membrane response to the hyperthermic challenge. In the immediate post hyperthermic period, this enhanced membrane stability will reduce the likelihood that a chemotherapeutic agent would enter the cell and produce cytotoxicity. Inactivation of cells by heat is largely a result of membrane inactivation, and there is a very sharp threshold at approximately 42 °C. All of the foregoing observations provide an explanation for the mechanism of interaction between hyperthermia and doxorubicin. Hyperthermic treatment results in an increase in cell membrane permeability which results in an increase in the intracellular concentration of doxorubicin for any given extracellular concentration of that drug at the time the hyperthermia is delivered when a temperature above 42 °C is achieved. Following administration of hyperthermia, however, synthesis of membrane stabilizing heat-shock proteins reduces the ratio of concentrations of intracellular vs. extracellular doxorubicin as is observed experimentally. For this reason, a rational protocol for the use of these two modalities in combination is to assure an adequate doxorubicin concentration in the tumor at the time hyperthermia is applied, and further, to assure that temperatures in excess of 42 °C are achieved with the hyperthermia treatment.

Another factor complicating the interaction of hyperthermia and chemotherapy is the relative structure of a tumor. Tumors have very heterogeneous histologies, with areas of necrosis, areas heavily infiltrated with inflammatory cells, and areas with structures that have the appearance of normal
tissue. Perfusion in these various areas is markedly different, and necrotic
regions of the tumor will be under perfused and not receive substantial drug
concentrations. However, these regions of the tumor cannot easily dissipate
heat and easily achieve high temperatures. Monitoring temperatures in these
areas is likely to result in an overestimation of the temperature in well
perfused regions of the tumor where a potentially therapeutic concentration
of the drug may exist. A corrollary to this effect of differences in perfusion is
that at high temperature, vascular collapse resulting in under-perfusion and
subsequent overheating and under-concentration of drug may occur. It has
been demonstrated that vascular collapse will certainly occur at temperatures above 44 °C. With the threshold of activation for a certain class of
drugs being at 42 °C, this leaves a very small therapeutic window for the
rational application of this combined modality.

Drugs which demonstrate a linear increase in biological effect with heat
are easier to use in rational treatment protocols. Any increase in temperature while the drug is present will produce an enhanced result in the heated
area. There is no need to assure reaching a threshold temperature and at the
same time not exceed a temperature which will certainly result in vascular
collapse in the heated area. Drugs in this category include the simple alkylators as well as the bifunctional alkylators along with some agents having
additional properties such as mitomycin-C and cisplatin. No studies have
demonstrated a time dependence for the administration of hyperthermia
and these drugs, so that a membrane effect is not readily postulated. There
is some suggestion that at least for cytoxan, which must be converted by
microsomal metabolism to an active alkylating moiety, this conversion is
increased at higher temperatures within the cells of the tumor. However, the
only known source of the active metabolite of patients is the liver and this is
not generally in the hyperthermia field except when it is the subject of the
treatment. On the other hand, simple first order thermodynamic effects on
chemical kinetics would be sufficient to explain the observed results with
this class of drugs, and studies need to be performed to demonstrate this
proposition.

The group of drugs which become cytotoxic at elevated temperature perhaps offers the most potential for study. Simple ethyl alcohol falls in this
category, as do the 'caine' anesthetics, but the best studied drug is amphotericin-B. Many other drugs which have not been studied are potential candidates for this class of substances and could provide an extraordinarily
powerful therapeutic armamentarium. Drugs free of dose-limiting toxicity at
reasonable concentrations which become cytotoxic only in the heated vol-

ume would allow extended and repeated treatments without concern for normal tissue tolerance. Unfortunately, amphotericin-B is quite toxic in its own right and cannot be used with impunity. Lidocaine has acute cardiac toxicity when administered systemically and this limits its use as a hyperthermic potentiator. Both of these agents are membrane active drugs and it is likely that this bears on the mechanism of action which results in cytotoxicity in the presence of hyperthermia. Therefore, an avenue of research examining other potentially membrane active drugs could result in finding an appropriate combination with therapeutic efficacy within the heated volume but few side effects within euthermic areas of the patient.

In vivo studies of combined hyperthermia and chemotherapy have been limited to animal models. Marmor [25] demonstrated synergy in a rat model with the simultaneous administration of local microwave hyperthermia and Thio-tepa. Marmor et al. [26] were unable to show therapeutic advantage with either doxorubicin or bleomycin in a rat model when used with hyperthermia. On the other hand, Overgaard [27] did demonstrate an enhanced anti-tumor effect when doxorubicin was used in conjunction with hyperthermia at 41.5 °C.

Clinical studies today have been limited to ongoing pilot studies primarily using alkylating agents or cisplatin. The lack of a threshold temperature and the need for exquisite timing of the modalities have made these drugs the most likely to produce fruitful clinical results in initial studies. As the results of such studies become available in the general literature, rational multi-institutional protocols can be designed and carried out in an attempt to demonstrate those clinical situations in which this combination of modalities is likely to be of definite benefit.

Hyperthermic techniques

Several approaches to the delivery of hyperthermia have been proposed, attempted and even commercially developed. Generally speaking, the electronically based methods have found more favor than direct application of heat, whether by water bath, heated air jet or even extracorporal perfusion heating. The electronic methods of hyperthermia application fall into three broad categories. First is RF energy, defined as the use of electromagnetic radiation in the range from 5–50 MHz. The second is microwave hyperthermia, which is generally considered to be electromagnetic radiation in the frequency range of 300 to 3000 MHz. Finally, ultrasound is used wherein the basic modality is high-frequency mechanical vibrational interaction with tissue; however, this vibration is electronically generated and the frequencies commonly used range from 1 to 3 MHz.

Ultrasonic hyperthermia is a relatively new technique, though the modality has been used extensively for diathermy in extremities by physical therapists. The primary limitation of this modality is the inability of the sonic energy to pass across areas of high mechanical impedance such as gas or air-filled structures. Regions of low impedance such as bone reflect the energy, blocking its application to deeper structures.

When comparing the direct application of electromagnetic energy to tissue, the very real difference in characteristics between RF and microwave radiation are a direct result of their respective wavelengths. Microwave radiation characteristically has a wavelength in air of the order of 30 cm; its wavelength in tissue is significantly less. For this reason, both the electric and the magnetic components can be transmitted with the usual ratio in the field intensities found when such radiation is transmitted in free space. The depth of penetration of microwave radiation is directly proportional to its wavelength in the tissue being treated.

A formidable problem related to the study of local tumor hyperthermia is that of temperature measurement in the lesion. If standard thermocouples or thermistors are to be used, then they must be inserted into the lesion. To determine a temperature profile, it is necessary to have the probe inserted as nearly as possible into the center of the lesion and near its deepest aspect. Also, it is desirable to have a probe at the periphery of the lesion, at least for some of the treatments, to determine temperature uniformity. Additionally, a thermocouple or thermistor inserted intradermally will allow skin temperature to be monitored.

While there is considerable difficulty characterizing the techniques for deep hyperthermia, superficial hyperthermia delivered by microwave or ultrasonic techniques is relatively well developed and in routine use in several centers. In fact, BSD Medical Corporation and Clinitherm Corporation have received pre-market approval to marked their equipment for superficial hyperthermia, both of which operate at microwave frequencies. The use of such units is no longer felt to be experimental.

Clinical trials

Clinical use of radiotherapy and hyperthermia in the treatment of patients has been reported sporadically for more than 80 years [28–30]. This treatment has employed either artificial fever or local application of heat through contact thermal sources. The occasionally good anecdotal response obtained suggested it was appropriate to continue to investigate this combination of therapies when no other accepted treatment alternative existed. As encouraging results continued to be obtained, certain investigators have begun to explore systematically the treatment of malignant tumors using this combination of modalities.

Kim et al. [31–35] reported several studies where hyperthermia was combined with radiotherapy to treat malignancies including Kaposi's sarcoma, mycosis fungoides, histiocytic lymphoma, synovial cell sarcoma, and multiple malignant cutaneous melanomas. Heat treatment was by contact hyperthermia or radiofrequency methods using 27 MHz and 13.5 MHz with magnetic induction coupling. In one group of patients they found that radiation alone produced 30 % responses, whereas, radiation and heat produced 50 % responses. In another group of patients they found radiation produced 50 % responses, while radiation and hyperthermia produced as high as an 80 % response rate.

Hornback et al. [36–38] reported on clinical trials using 433 MHz microwave sources to heat patients in conjunction with radiation therapy. Several of these patients had been previously treated, and in these patients 3000 rad of ionizing radiation was felt to be a maximum safe dose. In patients who had not previously been radiated, they treated to 6000 rad. Various histologies, including squamous cell carcinoma of the head and neck, sarcomas, adenocarcinomas and melanoma were treated. For an initial group of 21 patients who completed therapy, an 80 % response rate was obtained. In a later study, 72 patients were treated, representing 33 squamous cell carcinomas, 25 adenocarcinomas, three melanomas and 11 other lesions. These were divided into 12 patients treated with radiation plus heat, while 60 patients were treated with heat followed by radiation. Of the 12, 11 had complete responses, one had a partial response. Among the 60, there were 44 complete responders and 26 partial responders, with only two non-responders. No toxicity, other than the physiologic stress of the hyperthermia treatment itself, was associated with this group's study.

Marmor et al. [39, 40] used ultrasound hyperthermia in combination with radiotherapy to treat superficial lesions. Some were treated with radiotherapy, and some were treated with a combination of hyperthermia and radiotherapy. The end point of this study was to determine which arm produced superior response. Of 15 treatment sequences, seven showed an increased response with combination therapy, while only one showed a superior response to radiotherapy alone. Seven of the 15 showed no difference. Approximately 20 % of the patients exhibited significant pain from the ultrasound therapy, approximately 16 % developed superficial burns, and two patients exhibited an enhanced reaction over and above that caused by the radiation. However, this reaction ultimately healed.

U et al. [41] studied microwave-induced local hyperthermia in combination with radiotherapy. Altogether, 19 patients were treated, and they obtained 14 complete responders when a thermal dose of 42–44 °C for 40–50 min was delivered 10 min after radiotherapy. Microwave absorption in tissue was the method of delivery of the hyperthermia by these investigators.

Fazekas [43] studied the effects of localized hyperthermia with radiotherapy for superficial recurrent carcinoma. The thermal dose for this group was 43.5 °C for 40 min. Forty-six patients with 59 lesions were treated; 34 completed treatment as planned. Half of these had chest wall lesions; seven were melanoma and the rest were combinations of metastatic lesions to the skin. Twelve had complete responses, nine had partial responses, nine had no response. Hyperthermia in this study was delivered using 2450 MHz microwaves; and the documented shallow penetration of this energy could have resulted in the relatively lower response rate reported in this study.

Manning et al. [36] reported on the results of a phase 1 trial employing either hyperthermia alone or in combination with external beam or interstitial radiotherapy in a variety of patients. Heat delivery was either externally applied microwave hyperthermia or via interstitial antennae implanted in the tumor and activated with RF energy. Tumors included squamous cell carcinomas, adenocarcinomas, melanomas and sarcomas. Among patients treated with hyperthermia alone, there was an 18% complete response rate, 27% partial response rate and 55% non-responders. When radiation therapy was given and the doses ranged from 500–6000 rad, depending on previous treatment, the complete response rate increased to 27% with 53% exhibiting partial responses at the end of treatment. Only 20% were non-responders. When the interstitially applied hyperthermia and radiotherapy patients were examined, there was a 71% complete response rate with 29% partial responders and no non-responders. Their complication rate included one severe burn, several blisters, and various sequelae of rapid tumor regression, such as the production of a vaginorectal fistula.

The preceding studies of patients with advanced disease used radiotherapeutic regimens atypical of definitive treatment of primary cancer. Reported results only suggested improved efficacy with the combination therapy composed with that expected from palliative radiation alone as typically used in this advanced patient population. Encouraged by these early results, studies were undertaken on a pilot basis to demonstrate increased efficacy from combination therapy using internal controls. Archangeli et al. [44, 45] studied patients with two lesions, presumably of the same histology but spacially separated. These patients had their entire disease burden treated by radiation therapy with hyperthermia added to one lesion in an effort to demonstrate improved efficacy for the combination treatment in that lesion. However, unusual schedules of radiation therapy were used, some patients being treated with infrequent large fractions of radiation while others were treated with multiple daily fractions. All four reported schedules demonstrated an improved efficacy. The internal controls in this study demonstrated improved efficacy for hyperthermia; however, the response of the control lesions could not be compared with that achieved in historical series due to the unusual schedule of radiation therapy employed. The studies of

Scott et al. [46, 47] employed conventional schedules of radiation therapy, 60–66 Gy in 2 Gy daily fractions 5 days per week. A clear advantage was demonstrated in the lesions treated with combination hyperthermia and radiotherapy. However, due to progression in the control lesions within the patient population, no survival benefit could be demonstrated. The extended follow-up study by Scott et al. [47], while unable to demonstrate survival advantage, did demonstrate a significantly reduced recurrence rate for combination therapy as compared with that observed in the lesions treated with radiotherapy alone.

The largest and most comprehensive clinical trial is being completed by the Radiation Therapy Oncology Group. This study was activated in August, 1981 with the two objectives of determining the safety of the addition of superficial hyperthermia to conventionally accepted definitive radiotherapy and to attempt to demonstrate enhanced efficacy of the combination by comparison with historical controls. The study was open to institutions which had appropriate equipment to treat malignant tumors located within 3–4 cm of the skin surface. All patient treatments have been accomplished with externally applied microwave hyperthermia.

In evaluating this ongoing study, it is felt that the first objective has been achieved. Complications which have resulted from combination therapy are divided into three categories: (1) thermal burns or blisters, (2) ulceration or necrosis of skin secondary to hyperthermia or secondary to rapid tumor response and finally (3) an enhanced radiation reaction secondary to the hyperthermia where this could be spacially determined. Thermal burns occurred in approximately 10% of patients, and healed uneventfully in all patients. Skin ulceration, scored as a treatment complication or a result of rapid tumor response, occurred in approximately 10% of patients. While healing was delayed, probably secondary to the radiation therapy being applied, only one patient suffered from this complication 9 months post therapy. At 12 months and beyond no patients suffered from skin ulceration. There was no enhanced reaction in the radiation field secondary to the hyperthermia. All patients were treated with a radiation field larger than the hyperthermia field and in no case was an excess reaction noted within the demarcated hyperthermia field.

In assessing the efficacy of treatment it is important to recognize that protocol eligibility required that patients have disease of an advanced nature for which no other therapy would likely be of benefit. Approximately 85 patients completed therapy and were available for 3-month follow-up. Complete response was obtained in 78% of those study lesions at the 3-month follow-up. At 9 months, approximately 70% of lesions were complete responders and 70% of the ovarall patient group were survivors. This response and survival relationship eventually approached 60% for both complete responders and survivors and has become horizontal at about 18 months. A summary of the incidence and time course of complications and treatment efficacy is illustrated in Table 1.

Further analysis of this patient group has identified two disease sites for which presence of a superficial malignancy can have a negative impact on survival. These two sites are carcinoma of the head and neck region, where presence or absence of metastatic lymph nodes is an important prognostic factor; and chest wall recurrences of adenocarcinoma of the breast. These sites will be individually discussed in more detail.

Head and neck cancer

Of the 85 patients with a minimum 3-month follow-up there were 22 who presented with advanced, node positive, head and neck cancer. These patients were referred for radiotherapy due to inoperability secondary to the nature or extent of their disease and/or to medical contraindications to a major surgical procedure.

A recent report by Griffin et al. [48] provides a comprehensive analysis using an extensive data base of this class of patients. Nine-hundred and ninety-seven patients with the same contraindications to surgical treatment of their head and neck cancer were studied to elucidate prognostic factors which would allow prediction of success or failure in treating this class of patient. Multivariate analysis using sophisticated statistical techniques revealed that four factors were important in predicting response to definitive radiation therapy. These included the T-stage and N-stage size of the primary tumor (T-stage), the involvement of regional nodes (N-stage), the site of the primary tumor, and the patient's performance (Karnofsky) status at presentation. For the 997 patients analyzed, the predicted/observed ratio for each prognostic factor independently agreed to within at least 1%. An equation was developed with prediction accuracy of disease clearance better than 1%.

Table 1.

Follow-up (months)	Complete response (%)	Survival*	Thermal burns*	Skin ulcers*
3	76	100	10	10
6	88	90	–	10
12	72	72	–	–
18	70	70	–	–
24	69	69	–	–

* Percentage of patients completing therapy.

The 22 patients who completed hyperthermia and radiotherapy were analyzed and the probability of clearing disease with radiotherapy alone in each patient was calculated. Once the probabilities of clearance for each patient were known, they were averaged. The overall average calculated probability of disease clearance from the use of radiotherapy alone was 56%. The rate of clearance actually observed for this group of patients was 77%. When chi-squared analysis is used with one degree of freedom, such that the dependent variable is the presence or absence of hyperthermia and the independent variable the expected clearance of disease, this difference is significant at the 95% confidence level.

This difference between predicted and observed clearance refers to the entire group of patients. A case-by-case analysis was performed in an attempt to identify the prognostic factor whose influence from hyperthermia could account for these results.

All of these patients were treated using superficial microwave hyperthermia so the extent of the treatment depth was such that only the involved lymph nodes were likely to have received effective hyperthermia. For this reason, our analysis was modified by the assumption that the enhanced clearance observed with hyperthermia was entirely a result of eliminating the negative prognostic significance of their positive cervical lymph nodes. To analyze this assumption, the probability of disease clearance for each patient on a case-by-case basis was recalculated assuming that each one was indeed node negative in spite of his actual nodal status. This second set of probabilities was then averaged and the recalculated overall probability of disease clearance was 71%, statistically no different from the actual 77% observed.

At this juncture, we must address the question as to whether this exercise results in a strong case-by-case correlation between expected and observed clearance. When the recalculated probability of clearance for a given case was materially less than 50%, clinical failure was the rule, and when above 50% success was the rule. Scattered around the recalculated 50% mark is a sporadic observation of success and failure. While outstanding correlation was obtained, it must be emphasized that this correlation represents an exercise in mathematical analysis and does not demonstrate cause and effect. No demonstration or representation is made in this report that all nodal disease was indeed cleared, and in fact, at this time that data is not yet available. However, to the extent that node positive disease resulted in a detrimental prognostic factor to the probability of clearing the patient's disease, the addition of superficial microwave hyperthermia to these positive neck nodes negated that detrimental effect on a statistical basis.

Chest wall recurrences of adenocarcinomas of the breast

Several studies have demonstrated that many patients who fail local modality treatment, in particular surgical management of breast cancer, fail locally in the chest wall and proximal draining lymphatics without evidence of distant disease. This is all the more likely in patients failing adjuvant chemotherapy. It has been widely accepted that a local recurrence of adenocarcinoma of the breast automatically implies systemic disease. However, a certain fraction of patients appears to present with only locoregional recurrence. Three published series are used to demonstrate that up to two-thirds of patients with recurrent adenocarcinoma of the breast fall into this category (Table 2). These patients are typically treated with either re-excision, when that is possible, and/or radiation therapy in the event of inoperability or incomplete resection. It has been accepted that treatment of chest wall recurrence yielded only an improved quality of life as survival was not likely to be influenced by local control in the face of the systemic disease which was presumed to exist. Nonetheless, the recent report by Beck et al. [49] demonstrated that in those patients in whom complete control of the local disease was obtained, whether by re-excision or radiotherapy, a significantly improved survival at 5 years was demonstrated over those in whom local control was not obtained (Table 3). When the response to conventional

Table 2. Adenocarcinoma of the breast recurrent to the chest wall.

Local/regional recurrence only	L-R recurrence plus systemic disease	Series
121	54	Beck et al. [49]
124	73	Toonkel et al. [51]
178	84	Bedwinek et al. [52]
215	—	Chy et al. [53]

Table 3. Recurrent adenocarcinoma of the breast recurrent to the chest wall.

5-year survival				
Complete response	Overall	Partial/no response		Series
63%	38%	24%	$p < 0.01$	Beck et al. [49]
26%	36%	9%		Chu et al. [53]
				Toonkel et al. [51]
				Bedwinek et al. [52]

management (primarily radiation therapy), for 425 patients reported in recent literature is examined, one finds that the best complete response rate reported for any group is about 60–65%. In the 24–36-month follow-up period the retained complete response rate falls to approximately 30–35%. Against that background, similar patients, treated with combined hyperthermia/radiotherapy are analyzed.

Thirty patients have been treated for recurrent adenocarcinoma of the breast using combination radiotherapy and hyperthermia. The complete response rate in the 3-month period is 87%. This compares favorably with the results from Scott et al. [47] reporting on a 24-patient series in which 94% obtained complete response. In the 24–36-month time period, the complete response rate in the 30 patients remained at 70% comparing favorably with the results of the series by Scott et al. where an 80% sustained response rate was maintained and that by Perez et al. [50] which reported a 71% sustained response rate. This data implies that not only does combination therapy result in an enhanced clearance of local recurrence of adenocarcinoma of the breast when compared with recent reports using radiotherapy alone, but more dramatically these responses are sustained in extended follow-up (see Table 4).

Reexamination of the paired lesion data of Scott et al. [47] reveals that the risk for recurrence in the lesions treated with conventional radiation only was approximately 0.2 recurrences per lesion per 6-month period. When lesions treated with combination therapy were analyzed the recurrent rate was found to be 0.03 per lesion per 6 months. This was a statistically significant difference. If these recurrence rates are applied to the literature surveys cited, one would expect that half of the responses obtained by radiation therapy would have recurred within a 30-month period and indeed one can infer such a recurrence rate from a review of the recently published literature. Moreover, one would expect approximately 15% of lesions treated with combination therapy to have recurred and indeed the

Table 4. Adenocarcinoma of the breast recurrent to the chest wall.

	Radiation series [49, 51–53]	Radiation alone control lesions [46, 47]	Radiation plus hyperthermia [46, 47, 50])
Best complete response rate	193/290 (66%)	14/24 (58%)	65/84 (77%)
24–86-month retained complete response rate	144/415 (35%)	4/10 (40%)	18/25 (72%)

results of the 84 patients cited demonstrate such a recurrence rate in the 24–36-month time frame.

How does this implied improvement in local control, both in the immediate post therapy period as well as the follow-up period, relate to survival? We can again examine the reported results found in a literature review of four series; those by Beck et al. [49], Toonkel et al. [51], Bedwinek et al. [52], and Chu et al. [53]. The overall survival in these series reflected a survival following recurrence of adenocarcinoma of the chestwall of approximately 30% at 5 years, or slightly less than the sustained local response rate. In contrast, patients followed to 24–30 months treated with combination therapy have a survival of approximately 70% which is identical with the sustained control rate. For whatever reason the survival for patients treated with radiation therapy alone, with or without surgical or hormonal management, is nearly the same as the local control rates reported in those series (see Table 5). Again, as with cancers of the head and neck, a strong suggestion for overall improvement in tumor control as well as survival is suggested by this study.

Conclusion

In vitro and *in vivo* studies demonstrate that hyperthermia is cytoxic; is synergistic with radiation therapy, and has the potential for synergy with chemotherapy. Early clinical studies have confirmed an enhanced response rate for tumors treated with combination radiation therapy and superficial hyperthermia. These studies have further demonstrated that this combination can be used with acceptable toxicity. Acceptance of these results has resulted in the U.S. Food and Drug Administration granting pre-market approval to certain manufacturers, removing the 'investigational' label from this modality. Recent clinical studies have shown that the enhanced response rate from combined therapy is durable, indeed more durable than that obtained from radiotherapy alone. Moreover, tumor sites have been

Table 5. Adenocarcinoma of the breast recurrent to the chest wall – correlation of local control with survival.

	Radiation series (425 pts)	Radiation plus hyperthermia (42 pts)
Sustained 24–36-month complete response	34.8%	72%
3–5-year survival	32.7%	67%

identified where superficial disease can have a negative impact on patient survival. In these sites, an improved durable response rate is likely to result in real survival benefit to the patient.

The multiplicity and complexity of the interactions demonstrated between hyperthermia and chemotherapy hold out the promise for a clinical strategy with even greater therapeutic gain than achieved with radiotherapy.

References

1. Busch W. 1866. Bever den einfluss welihen heftigere Erysipeln Zuweilen auf organistierte neubildungen ausuhen. Verhandl Naturh Preuss Rein Westphal 23:28.
2. Coley WB. 1893. The treatment of malignant tumors by repeated innoculations of erysipelas – with a report of 10 original cases. Am J Med Sci 105:487.
3. Warren S. 1935. Preliminary study of the effect of artificial fever upon hopeless tumor cases. Am J Roentenol 33:75.
4. Gerwick LE, Gillette EL, Dewey WC. 1975. Effect of heat and radiation on synchronous Chinese hamster cells: killing and repair. Rad Res 64:611.
5. Ben-Hur E, Bronk BV, Elkind MM. 1972. Thermally enhanced radioresponse of cultured Chinese hamster cells. Nature 238:209.
6. Ben-Hur E, Elkind MM, Bronk BV. 1974. Thermally enhanced radioresponse of cultures Chinese hamster cells: inhibition of repair of sublethal damage and enhancement of lethal damage. Rad Res 58:38.
7. Dewey WC, Throll DE, Gillette EC. 1977. Hyperthermia and radiation-a selective thermal effect on chronically hypoxic tumor cells *in vivo*. Int J Rad Onc Biol Phys. 2:99.
8. Freeman ML, Holakan EV, Highfield DP, Raaphorst GP, Spiro IJ, Dewey WC. 1981. The effect of pH on hyperthermia and X-ray induced cell killing. Int J Rad Onc Biol Phys 7:211.
9. Dewhirst MW, Ozimek EJ, Gross J, Vetos TC. 1980. Will hyperthermia conquer the elusive hypoxic cell?: implications of heat effects on tumor and normal tissue microcirculation. Radiology 137:811.
10. Stewart JR, Gibbs FA, Lehman CM, Peck JW, Egger MJ. 1983. Change in the *in vivo* hyperthermic response resulting from the metabolic effects of temporary vascular occlusion. Int J Rad Onc Biol Phys 9:197.
11. Sapareto SA, Hopwood LE, Dewey WC, Raju MR, Gray JW. 1978. Effects of hyperthermia on survival and progression of Chinese hamster ovary cells. Cancer Res 38:393.
12. Robinson JE, Wizenberg MJ, McCready WA. 1974. Radiation and hyperthermia response of normal tissue in situ. *Radiology 113*:195.
13. Overgaard J. 1980. Simultaneous and sequential hyperthermia and radiation treatment of an experimental tumor and its surrounding normal tissue *in vivo*. Int J Rad Onc Biol Phys 6:1507.
14. Emami B, Nussbaum GH, Hahn N, Pio AJ, Dritschilo A, Quimby F. 1981. Histopathological study on the effects of hyperthermia on microvasculature. Int J Rad Onc Bio Phys 7:343.
15. Emami B, Nussbaum GH, Ten Haken RK, Hughes WL. 1980. Physiological effects of hyperthermia: response of capillary blood flow and structure to local tumor heating. Radiology 137:805.
16. Eddy HA, Chmielewski G. 1982. Effect of hyperthermia, radiation and adriamycin combinations on tumor vascular function, Int J Rad Onc Biol Phys 8:1167.

17. Eddy HA. 1980. Alterations in tumor microvasculature during hyperthermia. Radiology 137:515.
18. Song CW, Kang MS, Rhec JG, Levitt SH. 1980. The effect of hyperthermia on vascular function, pH and cell survival. Radiology 137:795.
19. Freeman ML, Boone MCM, Ensley BA, Gillette, EL. 1981. The influence of environmental pH on the interaction and repair of heat and radiation damages. Int J Rad Onc Biol Phys 7:761.
20. Urano M, Rice LC, Montoya V. 1982. Studies on fractionated hyperthermia in experimental animal systems II response of murine tumors to 2 or more doses. Int J Rad Onc Biol Phys 8:227.
21. Spiro IJ, Sapareto SA, Raaphorst GP, Dewey WC. 1982. The effect of chronic and acute heat conditioning on the development of thermal tolerance. Int J Rad Onc Biol Phys 8:53.
22. Landry J, Chretien P, Bernier D, Nichole LM, Marceau N, Tonguay rm. 1982. Thermotolerance and heat shock proteins induced by hyperthermia in rat live cells. Int J Rad Onc Biol Phys 8:59.
23. Li GC, Peterson NS, Mitchell HK. 1982. Induced thermal olerance and heat shock protein synthesis in Chinese hamster ovary cells Int J Rad Onc Biol Phys 8:63.
24. Hahn GM, Strande DP. 1976. Cytotoxic effects of hyperthermia and Adriamycin on Chinese hamster cells. J Natl Cancer Inst 57:1063–1067.
25. Marmor JB. 1979. Interactions of hyperthermia and chemotherapy in animals. Cancer Res 39:2269–2276.
26. Marmor JB, Kozak D, Hahn GM. 1979. Effects of systemic bleomycin or Adriamycin with local hyperthermia on primary tumor and lung metastases. Cancer Treat Rep 63:1279–1290.
27. Overgaard J. 1976. Combined Adriamycin and hyperthermia treatment of a murine Mammary carcinoma *in vivo*. Cancer Res 36:3077–3081.
28. Rohdenburg Gl, Prime F. 1921. Effect of combination radiation and heat on neoplasmas. Arch Surg 2:116.
29. Doub H. 1935. Osteogenic sarcoma of clavicle treated with radiation and fever Therapy. Radiology 25:355.
30. Allen FM. 1955. Biological modification of effects of roentgen rays. II high temperature and related factors. Am J Roentgenol 73:836.
31. Kim JH, Hahn EW, Tokita N, Nisce LZ. 1977. Local tumor hyperthermia in combination with radiotherapy 1. malignant cutaneous lesions. Cancer 40:161.
32. Kim JH, Hahn EW, Tokita N. 1978. Combination hyperthermia and radiation therapy for cutaneous malignant melanoma. Cancer 41:2143.
33. Rofstad EK, Brustad T. 1982. Effect of Hyperthermia on human melanoma cells heated either as solid tumors in athymic nude mise or *in vitro*. Cancer 50:1304.
34. Kim JH, Hahn EW, Tokita N. 1978. Combination hyperthermia and radiation therapy for cutaneous malignant melanoma. Cancer 41:2143.
35. Kim JH, Hahn EW, Ahmed SA. 1982. Combination hyperthermia and radiation therapy for malignant melanoma. Cancer 50:478.
36. Hornback NB, Shupe RE, Shidnia H, Joe BT, Sayoc E, Marshall C. 1977. Preliminary clinical results of combined 433 MHz microwave therapy and radiation therapy on patients with advanced cancer. Cancer 40:2854.
37. Hornback HB, Shupe R, Shidnig H, Joe BT, Sayoc E, George R, Marschall C. 1979. Radiation and microwave therapy in the treatment of advanced cancer. Radiology 130:459.
38. Hornback NB, Shidnia H, Shupe RE, Reddy s, Marshall C, Baker R: 1980. Results comparing hyperthermic and radiation vs. radiation alone in treatment of 79 patients with stage III-B carcinoma of uterine cervix. Int J Rad Onc Biol Phys 6:1384.

39. Marmor JB, Pounds D, Postic TB, Hahn G. 1979. Treatment of superficial human neoplasms by local hyperthermia induced by ultrasound. Cancer 43:188.
40. Marmor JB, Hahn GM. 1980. Combined radiation and hyperthermia in superficial human
tumors. Cancer 46:1986.
41. U R, Noell KT, Woodward KT, Wordes BT, Fishburn RI, Miller LS. 1980. Microwave-
induced local hyperthermia incombination with radiotherapy of human malignant tumors.
Cancer 45:638.
42. Fazelas JT, Nerlinger RE. 1980. Localized hyperthermia adjuvant to irradiation in superficial recurrent carcinomas: a preliminary report on 46 patients. Int J Rad Onc Biol Phys
7:1457.
43. Manning MR, Cetas tC, Miller RC, Oleson JR, Conner WG, Gerner EW. 1982. Clinical
hyperthermia: results of phase I trial employing hyperthermia alone or in combination with
external beam or interstitial radiotherapy. Cancer 49:205.
44. Arcangeli G, Barni E, Cividalli A, Mauro F, Moulli D, Nervi C, Spano M, Tabocchini A.
1980. Effectiveness of microwave hyperthermia combined with ionizing radiation: clinical
results on neck node metastasis, Int J Rad Onc Biol Phys 6:43.
45. Arcangeli G, Cividalli A, Nervi C, Creton G, Lovisolo G, Mauro F. 1983. Tumor control
and therapeutic gain with different schedules of combined radiotherapy and local external
hyperthermia in human cancer, Int J Rad Onc Biol Phys 9:1125.
46. Scott RS, Johnson RJR, Kowal H, Krishnamsetty Rm. Story K, Clay L. 1982. Hyperthermia
in combination with radiotherapy: a review of five years experience in the treatment of
superficial tumors. Int J Rad Onc Biol Phys 1327.
47. Scott RS, Johnson RJR, Storey KV, Clay L. 1984. Local hyperthermia in combination with
definitive radiotherapy: Increased tumor clearance, reduced recurrence rate in extended fol-
lowup. Int J Rad Oncol Biol Phys 10:2119–2123.
48. Griffin TW, Pajak TF, Gillespie BW, Davis LW, Brady LW, Rubin P, Marcial VA. 1984.
Predicting the response of head and neck cancer to radiation therapy with a multivariate
modeling system: An analysis of the RTOG head and neck registry. Int J Radiat. Oncol Biol
Phys 10:481–487.
49. Beck, TM, Hart NE, Woodland DA, Smith CE. 1984. Local or regionally recurrent carcinoma of the breast: results of therapy in 121 patients. J Clin Oncol 1:400–405.
50. Perez CA, Nussbaum G, Emami B, Von Gerichten D. 1983. Clinical Results of irradiation
combined with local hyperthermia. Cancer 52:1597–1603.
51. Toonkel LM, Fix I, Jacobson LH, Wallach CB. 1983. The significance of local recurrence of
carcinoma of the breast. Int J Radiat Oncol Biol Phys 9:33–40.
52. Bedwinek JM, Fineberg B, Lee J, Ocwieza M. 1981. Analysis of failures following local
treatment of isolated local-regional recurrence of breast cancer Int J Radiat Oncol Biol Phys
7:581–585.
53. Chu FCH, Fong-Jen, L, Kim JH, Huh SH, Garmatis CJ. 1976. Locally recurrent carcinoma
of the breast. Results of radiation therapy. Cancer 37:2677–2681.

7. Neurosurgical options in cancer pain management

ROBERT E. HARBAUGH and RICHARD L. SAUNDERS

Abstract

For the great majority of patients with cancer, pain can be managed without neurosurgical intervention. However, for those patients for whom other therapy is unsuccessful, neurosurgery offers a wide array of procedures for decreasing or eliminating pain and suffering. This chapter presents a brief review of the neuroanatomy and neurochemistry of pain transmission. Neurosurgical options for cancer pain management are discussed with regard to indications, expected results and complications. This chapter is not meant to be an exhaustive review, but rather, a useful reference for the range of neurosurgical procedures available for the patient with cancer pain.

Neuroanatomy

A brief review of the neuroanatomy of pain transmission is necessary for the understanding of neurosurgical procedures. Starting peripherally, painful stimuli are recognized by conduction through poorly myelinated A-delta fibers (fast pain) and unmyelinated C fibers (slow pain). Fast pain is of brief duration, well localized, and generally does not produce suffering. Slow pain is diffuse, persistent, and frequently associated with affective and visceral responses. It is this slow, C-fiber mediated pain which is of most concern to the physician dealing with the cancer patient.

The cell body of the peripheral pain fiber lies in the dorsal root ganglion. Projections to the spinal cord enter via both the dorsal and ventral roots. At the area of entry of the dorsal nerve roots into the cord, most nociceptive fibers traverse the laterally placed Lissauer's tract and terminate in laminae 1, 2 and 5 of the dorsal horn gray matter.

Second order projection neurons arise from the dorsal horn. Lamina 1 cells project to many levels of the neuraxis, and the neuroanatomy and

Higby, DJ (ed), Issues in Supportive Care of Cancer Patients. ISBN 0-89838-816-3.
© *1986, Martinus Nijhoff Publishers, Boston. Printed in the Netherlands.*

neurophysiology are not well understood. Lamina 5 cells appear to be the major contributors to the spinothalamic system. After crossing the midline in the anterior white commisure, axons of these second order neurons project cephalad in the lateral quadrant of the cord as the lateral spinothalamic tract. It is, however, important to note that ipsilateral and ventral contralateral projections also exist. The extent to which these alternative spinothalamic projections are responsible for nociception is not fully documented.

The lateral spinothalamic tract is somatotopically organized with more cephalad areas of the body represented in the more medial and inferior aspects of the tract. Numerous fibers from the spinothalamic system terminate in the reticular formation of the brain stem as well as project to the intralaminar and ventroposterolateral nuclei of the thalamus. From these structures, projection to essentially every region of the neuraxis is possible.

The role of the cerebral cortex in pain perception, although obviously of importance for a thorough understanding of pain and suffering, is not well documented. Although cortical 'pain centers' have been postulated, specific anatomic-behavioral correlation is lacking.

Perhaps as important for pain perception as the ascending projection systems are the descending systems modulating nociception. Starting at the caudal diencephalon and extending throughout the medial brain stem are cells of origin for descending systems that diminish pain perception. These systems appear to project caudally via the dorsolateral funiculus of the spinal cord to synapse in the dorsal horn. Both the anatomy and physiology of this descending system are less well understood than the ascending projection systems.

Neurochemistry

Understanding of the physiology of pain perception has been greatly augmented by advances in neurochemistry. It is no longer reasonable to explain behavioral anatomic correlates without discussion of the various neurotransmitters and neuromodulators involved.

There is relatively good evidence that primary afferent nociceptive neurons release a peptide neurotransmitter, substance P, in the dorsal horn of the spinal cord. This release of substance P can be modified by the activity of dorsal horn interneurons using endogenous opioid transmitters or somatostatin and probably by the descending control systems employing dopamine, serotonin, and norepinephrine. A review of the interactions of these various neurotransmitters is beyond the scope of this chapter and would, at best, be speculative. However, neurotransmitter modulation at spinal cord or higher levels can have a profound effect on pain perception without producing neuroanatomic disruption.

In summary, the simple concept of dividing a pain pathway to produce permanent, satisfactory pain relief is long outdated. Present understanding of neuroanatomy and neurochemistry, although far more difficult to grasp, offers more options for neurosurgical manipulation of nociception.

Neurosurgical options

Neurosurgical interventions for cancer pain management can be categorized by the level of the neuraxis which is approached and by the type of manipulation performed. The intervention options discussed in the following sections are listed in Table 1.

Peripheral nerve or root sectioning

Indications and patient selection
For neurectomy or rhizotomy to be effective, pain must be well localized in the distribution of a specific spinal or cranial nerve or of a limited number of nerve roots. In addition, the functional consequences of denervation in a given area must be considered. These concerns effectively limit the applicability of neurectomy and rhizotomy.

Unilateral high cervical and facial pain may be adequately controlled by rhizotomy of the ipsilateral trigeminal, nervus intermedius, glossopharyn-

Table 1. Neurosurgical options for cancer pain management.

	Type of intervention		
Site of intervention	Destructive lesion	Electrical stimulation	Neurotransmitter manipulation
Primary afferents	Nerve or root section	—	—
Spinal cord	Cordotomy Myelotomy Root entry zone legions	Dorsal column stimulation	Intraspinal analgesics
Brain stem	Medullary tractotomy Mesencephalic and thalamic lesions	Periaqueductal or periventricular stimulation	Intraventricular analgesics
Cerebral hemispheres	Cingulotomy Lobotomy	—	—
Other	Hypophysectomy	—	—

geal, and upper vagal roots combined with high cervical rhizotomy. Although this is an extensive operative procedure, the results can be gratifying when other therapeutic attempts have failed.

Pain involving the limbs is generally not amenable to neurectomy or rhizotomy because of the severe functional consequences of denervation. If, however, the neural involvement by tumor is such that the limb is already nonfunctional, then rhizotomy may be acceptable.

Unilateral or bilateral trunkal pain can be addressed by rhizotomy. For chest and abdominal pain, section of both the dorsal and ventral roots is probably advised because of the primary afferent projections via the ventral roots. For pelvic pain, bilateral denervations will result in urinary and fecal incontinence and should be considered only as a last resort in patients who still have sphincter control. Unilateral sacral rhizotomy is not usually associated with incontinence.

Results

Short-term results of neurectomy or rhizotomy can be very gratifying, but long-term outcome is generally not as rewarding. Although accurate failure rates are difficult to obtain from the literature, it seems safe to say that the longer the survival the greater the failure rate.

Risks and complications

Open rhizotomy is a major neurosurgical procedure entailing laminectomy and/or craniectomy and the risks attendant to such intervention. A significant perioperative mortality can be anticipated in debilitated cancer patients. Morbidity secondary to cerebrospinal fluid (CSF) leaks, poor wound healing, and infection occurs particularly in patients who have undergone radiation therapy at the operative site.

In contrast to the above, chemical rhizolysis for patients with pelvic pain and incontinence can be accomplished at the bedside with minimal morbidity. For this restricted group of patients, chemical rhizotomy may be the safest, most expenditious therapy for cancer pain.

Cordotomy

Indications and patient selection

Anterolateral cordotomy, whether done as an open procedure or percutaneously, is based on interruption of the lateral spinothalamic fibers for pain control. In general, open cordotomy has been replaced by the percutaneous procedure and discussion is limited to the latter.

Cordotomy may be considered for pain below the mandible in any patient with documented adequate pulmonary function. Unilateral or staged bilateral procedures can be done under local anesthesia via a percutaneous C 1-2 approach with fluoroscopic control and radiofrequency generated lesions.

Results
Immediate and short-term results of cordotomy are quite good, with approximately 90% of patients reporting good or excellent pain relief. However, this figure drops to 60 and 40% after 1 and 2 years, respectively. Bilateral pain, requiring bilateral cordotomies, is not only more dangerous but does not seem to respond as well to the procedure.

Risks and complications
Complications of percutaneous cordotomy are related primarily to lesions induced in the spinal cord adjacent to the lateral spinothalamic tract. These include ipsilateral hemiparesis (permanent in about 3% of cases), ataxia (3% permanent), urinary incontinence (2% permanent), and sleep induced apnea (3% permanent). A perioperative mortality in the range of 10% has been reported, with most deaths not directly related to the operative procedure.

In summary, percutaneous cordotomy remains a relatively effective procedure for short-term pain control in cancer patients. It is almost certainly the safest and most widely used destructive neurosurgical procedure for cancer pain management.

Myelotomy

Indications and patient selection
Open microsurgical division of the anterior commissure, which interrupts second order projection fibers going to both lateral spinothalamic tracts, has been used for patients with bilateral or midline pain in the lower half of the body.

Results
Pain relief has been achieved in 60 to 70% of patients in the immediate postoperative period. As with all ablative procedures, the longer the survival the lower this percentage.

Risks and complications
The risks associated with major neurosurgical procedures apply to commissural myelotomy. Neurologic complications include numbness and paresthesias, poor motor control, and sphincter disturbance. It is not a widely used procedure.

Dorsal root entry zone lesions

Indications and patient selection
Dorsal root entry zone (DREZ) lesions have been employed primarily for patients with deafferentation pain secondary to trauma, but extensive use of this procedure in cancer pain patients has not been reported. At present it should probably be considered only in those cancer pain patients where deafferentiation is present (for example, brachial plexus deafferentation from tumor involvement or radiation). The procedure involves open lesioning of the DREZ and dorsal horn by radiofrequency or laser energy.

Results
Results of cancer patients treated by DREZ lesions are not available.

Risks and complications
DREZ lesions require a major neurosurgical procedure with its attendant risks. Ipsilateral leg weakness is the most common complication, although various proprioceptive and other sensory changes have been reported. DREZ lesions should probably not be considered as a standard neurosurgical procedure for cancer pain management until further information is available.

Medullary tractotomy

Indications and patient selection
The spinal nucleus of the fifth cranial nerve is the cranial counterpart of the spinal cord dorsal horn. Nociceptive fibers from the fifth, seventh, ninth, and tenth cranial nerves converge on this nucleus via the spinal tract of the fifth cranial nerve. Therefore, lesions of the spinal nucleus and tract of the fifth cranial nerve are used for patients with ipsilateral facial pain. Medullary tractotomy may be used with upper cervical rhizotomy for ipsilateral facial and upper cervical pain.

Results
A 75 to 85% acceptable pain relief response rate has been reported for cancer patients with this procedure. However, few reports on the effectiveness of medullary tractotomy have been published.

Risks and complications
Perioperative mortality of up to 20% has been reported in cancer patients. Ataxia, proprioceptive loss, dysarthria, dysesthesia, trophic ulcers, intractable hiccups, and Horner's syndrome have all been reported as neurologic complications of this medullary tractotomy.

Thalamotomy

Indications and patient selection
Cancer pain involving the face and upper extremity is most commonly considered for sterotactic ablative lesions of the thalamus. Although numerous lesion sites have been suggested, discussion here is limited to lesions of the mesencephalon and medial thalamic nuclei.

Results
Initial good pain relief is achieved in 65 to 85 % of cancer pain patients with mesencephalotomy or thalomotomy. As with all destructive lesions, this figure decreases with time.

Risks and complications
Diplopia, loss of upward gaze, distressing dysesthesias, confusion, dysphasia, hemiparesis, and dementia have been reported with these lesions. They remain experimental procedures for cancer pain management which are available at relatively few centers.

Cingulotomy

Although included for the sake of completeness, this procedure is now done infrequently for cancer pain patients. Bilateral cingulotomy may be used for relief of the fear and suffering accompanying chronic cancer pain. A 50 % positive short-term response has been documented. Headache, confusion, incontinence, and personality change are relatively frequent but usually transient postoperative findings.

Hypophysectomy

Indications and patient selection
Although used primarily in cases of metastatic breast and prostate cancer, pain relief has been reported following hypophysectomy in a wide variety of metastatic tumors. The mechanism by which pain relief occurs, even without regression of the disease, is unknown.

Results
Initial pain relief in 75 to 90 % of patients with metastatic breast and prostate cancer has been reported. This is significantly higher than the percentage of patients who achieve objective remission of their tumors. Long-term results of pain relief are not readily available.

Risks and complications

Transphenoidal hypophysectomy, although a major neurosurgical procedure, is usually well tolerated. Most patients will develop at least a transient diabetes insipidus postoperatively which may require antidiuretic hormone replacement therapy. Postoperative corticosteroid and thyroid hormone replacement therapy are mandatory. Hypophysectomy should probably be considered for pain control only in those patients with breast and prostate cancer where other measures have failed or a chance of objective remission exists.

Dorsal column stimulation

Included for the sake of completeness only, dorsal column stimulation is now rarely done for patients with cancer pain. Operative complications such as poor wound healing, skin erosion, and infection have been reported, as have electrical system failure, distressing paresthesias, and electrode migration. Retrospective studies have shown consistently poor response in patients with cancer pain.

Periaqueductal and periventricular stimulation

Indications and patient selection

Stereotactic electrode placement and electrical stimulation of the periventricular/periaqueductal gray matter for pain control have been done since 1972. Activation of descending serotonergic and noradrenergic modulatory pathways are thought to be responsible for stimulation mediated analgesia. Whether this stimulation uses an endogenous opiate intermediary for such activation is controversial. The procedure has been used primarily for patients with cancer pain involving the face, pharynx, throat, or perineal area.

Results

Short-term pain relief is produced in about 90% of patients. Long-term relief is significantly less, with figures of 60 to 80% expected.

Risks and complications

Surgical complications of electrode placement such as infection, diplopia, and leg weakness have been reported. Electrical system malfunction, electrode migrations, and broken wires have also occurred. Tolerance to stimulation has occurred in a few patients. This approach to cancer pain management remains experimental and is used at relatively few medical centers.

Intraspinal and intraventricular analgesics

Because our research is in this area of cancer pain management and because this type of therapy has rapidly become accepted at many institutions, this section is somewhat more inclusive than the rest of the chapter.

Background

Identification of endogenous opiates and their receptors in the central nervous system prompted investigations into pain management by manipulation of this system. Percutaneous catheters and implanted infusion devices have been used to apply opiate or other analgesic compounds at the spinal cord or intraventricular level. Local modulation has the potential advantage of being able to affect nociception without deleterious effects at other levels of the neuraxis. In addition, because intraspinal and intraventricular analgesic infusions do not require destruction of neural tissue, the neurologic side effects are usually minimal. This approach to cancer pain management is still in its infancy, and much exciting work is presently underway. Many questions about the optimum drug, site, and pattern of delivery remain to be answered.

Indications and patient selection

One advantage of intraspinal and intraventricular analgesic is their applicability to essentially any cancer pain patient. Anatomic localization of pain does not seem to be a major factor in response to treatment, although some studies suggest that neck and face pain may respond better to intraventricular than to intraspinal narcotics. Because catheter placement is a relatively minor neurosurgical procedure, most patients can readily withstand the operative procedure. Patients who have shown no response to systemic narcotics are not likely to be responsive to central nervous system delivery of the same compounds.

Results

Short-term results of intraspinal and intraventricular analgesics in patients with cancer pain have been very good. However, analgesic procedures become less effective the longer the patient survives. Increased dosage of narcotics become necessary to maintain adequate analgesia paralleling the well-known but poorly understood phenomenon of narcotic tolerance with systemic administration. This phenomenon has been the major obstacle in attaining adequate analgesia with intraspinal and intraventricular narcotics. Various manipulations have been used to overcome this problem. Narcotic drug holidays, with analgesia maintained by epidural lidocaine and withdrawal minimized by clonidine, have occasionally been successful. The use of intraspinal adrenergic agonists for analgesia while narcotic infusion is discontinued is also being investigated. However, at present, no wholly successful approach to the problem of narcotic tolerance is available.

Risks and complications
Risks of intraspinal and intraventricular analgesia can be divided into risks of the operative procedure and risks of drug infusion. Catheter placement has a small risk of hemorrhage and infection. The problem of delayed sepsis is minimal with totally implantable systems. Percutaneous catheters represent a persistent site for infection, which increases incrementally with the duration of treatment.

Risks of narcotic drug infusion include apnea, nausea, pruritis, and urinary retention. Apnea has been observed only with bolus narcotic administration and usually occurs within six hours of drug delivery. This potentially fatal complication can occur as late as 24 hours after an intraspinal bolus and is rapidly reversed by intravenous administration of naloxone. Although experience with intraspinal adrenergic agonists for analgesia is limited, the only documented side effect to date is hypotension.

Summary

The chapter does not represent an exhaustive review of the neurosurgical procedures available for cancer pain management. However, it serves as a starting reference which outlines the wide range of neurosurgical interventions available for chronic pain.

In general, neurosurgical management of chronic pain seems to be moving away from the destruction lesions of the nervous system and toward more sophisticated neurochemical and electrical manipulation of nociceptive pathways. Experience has shown that pain conduction pathways are numerous and resilient. No single lesion is likely to produce permanent adequate analgesia, unless the patient's survival is relatively brief. This fact, in conjunction with the neurologic morbidity to be expected with any destructive lesion, makes destructive neurosurgery .ess palatable in an era when other modalities are available.

The optimum pain control procedure would produce permanent, absolute pain relief without interfering with any other nervous system functions. Such a procedure is not available today but is now at least a foreseeable goal.

References

1. Brodal A. 1981. Neurological Anatomy in Relation to Clinical Medicine. Oxford University Press, New York, pp 1953.
2. Coggeshall RE. Neurosurgery 4:443–448.
3. Coombs DW, Saunders RL. 1985. Intraspinal infusion of narcotic drugs. In: Neurosurgery Wilkins RH, Rengachary SS (eds), MacGraw-Hill, New York, pp 2390–2397.
4. Coombs DW, Saunders RL, Gaylor MS et al. 1983. Relief of continuous chronic pain by intraspinal narcotics infusion via and implanted reservoir. JAMA 250:2335–2339.
5. Harbaugh RE, Coombs DW, Saunders RL et al. 1982. Implanted continuous epidural morphine infusion system: Preliminary report. J Neurosurg 56:803–806.
6. King RB. 1977. Anterior commissurotomy for intractable pain. J Neurosurg 47:7–11.
7. Leavans ME, Hill CS, Cech DA et al. 1982. Intrathecal and intraventricular morphine for pain in cancer patients: Initial study. J Neurosurg 56:241–245.
8. Loeser JD. 1972. Dorsal rhizotomy for the relief of chronic pain. J Neurosurg 36:745–750.
9. Nashold BS Jr, Crue JBL Jr. 1982. Stereotactic mesencephalotomy and trigeminal tractotomy. In: Neurological Surgery Youmans JR (ed). WB Saunders, Philadelphia, pp 3702–3716.
10. Nashold BS, Ostahl RH. 1979. Dorsal root entry zone lesions for pain relief. J Neurosurg 51:59–69.
11. Richardson DE, Akil H. 1977. Pain reduction by electrical brain stimulation in man. J Neurosurg 47:178–183, 184–194.
12. Rosomoff HL. 1974. Percutaneous radiofrequency cervical cordotomy for intractable pain. Adv Neurol 4:683–688.
13. Tindall GT, Ambrose SS, Christy JH et al. 1976. Hypophysectomy in the treatment of disseminated carcinoma of the breast and prostate gland. South Med J 69:579–587.
14. Watkins ES. The place of neurosurgery in the relief of intractable pain. In: Relief of Intractable Pain Swerdlow M (ed). Excerpta Medica, Amsterdam pp 21–58.
15. White JC, Sweet WH. 1969. Pain and the Neurosurgeon. A Forty-Year Experience. Charles C. Thomas, Springfield, Il, pp 1000.
16. Young RG. 1978. Evaluation of dorsal column stimulation in the treatment of chronic pain. Neurosurgery 3:373–379.

8. Pulmonary disease in the cancer patient

JOHN N. LANDIS

Introduction

Patients with cancer can develop numerous pulmonary problems during the management of their underlying disease. The spectrum of involvement can run from a totally unrelated pre-existing pulmonary process such as asthma or emphysema to complications of the primary cancer and its management. The major focus of this review is on common problems: diffuse infiltrative lung disease, pulmonary infection, and pleural effusions. This review should alert the clinician caring for the cancer patient to the possibilities of pulmonary involvement and the importance of establishing an early and definitive diagnosis if therapy is to be effective.

There are seven categories of pulmonary disease that can affect the cancer patient:
1. pre-existing pulmonary disease unrelated to malignancy;
2. pulmonary disease directly related to underlying malignant diseaseß
3. pulmonary disease caused by infection;
4. pulmonary disease associated with drug toxicity;
5. a new pulmonary process unrelated to malignancy;
6. extrapulmonary disease – pleural effusion;
7. any combination of the above.

The symptoms of lung disease in the cancer patient include combinations of fever, non-productive cough or dyspnea. The chest X-ray may be normal but is frequently abnormal with focal infiltrative, reticular, reticulo-nodular, and alveolar infiltrative patterns. However, these are rarely diagnostic. Gas exchange is usually altered by hypoxemia, and many patients are leukopenic and anemic. As a consequence of leukopenia, infections are common; as a consequence of anemia, oxygen carrying capacity is compromised. Although there are diagnostic measures to establish an etiologic mechanism, in 15% to 20% of cancer patients the cause of pulmonary abnormality remains undiagnosed at autospy [1]. Pulmonary infections are the commonest cause

Higby, DJ (ed), Issues in Supportive Care of Cancer Patients. ISBN 0-89838-816-3.
© *1986, Martinus Nijhoff Publishers, Boston. Printed in the Netherlands.*

of pulmonary disease in the cancer patient accounting for approximately
75% of the diagnostic problems [2].

Pre-existing pulmonary disease

These illnesses are usually recognized by a careful history, physical exam
and pulmonary functional assessment. If obstruction to airflow is found,
treatment should consist of aerosolized and/or oral bronchodilators, usually
in the form of theophylline or a beta 2 sympathomimetic aerosol. Treatment is monitored by theophylline blood levels, peak flows, and subjective
response. If the patient stops smoking, further loss of FEV_1 is usually less
than 50 cc per year [3]. A patient with forms of airflow obstruction, emphysema, chronic bronchitis and asthma may have exacerbations of airways
disease following treatment with chemotherapeutic agents and radiation.
For instance, mediastinal radiation for lung cancer may result in airway
edema. Certain drugs may exacerbate bronchospasm because of irritant
receptor mechanisms (aerosolized drugs such as cystiene and polymyxin
B) [4] or direct action (penicillin and aspirin) [5].

In addition to forms of chronic obstructive pulmonary disease, patients in
later stages of life frequently have coexisting ischemic heart disease which
can produce and mimic the same symptoms as pulmonary disease. The
most common symptom is dyspnea; the senstation of breathlessness usually
reflects disease of the airways, lung parenchyma, pulmonary vasculature or
adjacent surrounding structures such as the heart or lungs.

Although some patients present with asthma and emphysema and respond to bronchodilator therapy, the lung is most commonly affected directly by metastatic involvement or indirectly as a consequence of cancer therapy. The mortality directly related to pulmonary disease in cancer patients
approaches 50% [1, 6].

Pulmonary disease directly related to underlying malignant disease

Pulmonary disease can arise due to pulmonary metastases which occur in
one-third of patients who die of extra-pulmonary cancer. These lesions may
be totally asymptomatic at first and appreciated only by chest X-ray or CT
scan of the lung. Lesions metastatic to the lung frequently originate from
primary tumors of the colon, kidney, breast, thyroid and testicles. Sarcomas,
(commonly osteogenic) and melanomas occasionally metastasize to this site.
Presentation on chest X-ray can be as solitary or multiple discrete nodules,
lymphangitic spread, hilar or mediastinal lymph node involvement, or pleural seeding. These metastatic nodules must be distinguished from benign

processes such as infectious granulomata, rheumatoid nodules, Wegener's granulomatosis and nodular sarcoidosis. Therefore, needle aspiration, bronchoscopy and sputum cytology are helpful in diagnosing specific lesions. The availability of previous chest X-rays is especially helpful in determining whether a nodular lesion is new and can be useful in determining whether surgical intervention should be recommended [7]. In a large series that studied rate of tumor enlargement, it was noted that nodular lesions with doubling times of less than 20 days rarely benefited from surgery, but those with times of greater than 40 days had a favorable prognosis after resection of metastatic nodules. Five-year survivorship of 60% was seen in the latter group. Spontaneous resolution of pulmonary metastases has also been reported with resection of primary genitourinary tumors [8]. Pulmonary resection of metastatic lesions has been successful in selected patients with metastatic carcinoma from the colon, melanoma, breast and testes [9].

The prognosis from other forms of metastatic involvement is much worse. Intrapulmonary lymphangitic spread is rapidly terminal. This form of metastasis frequently occurs with adenocarcinomas. Common primary sites are lung, stomach, breast and pancreas [10]. Although the chest X-ray may be initially normal, an interstitial pattern with diffuse irregular and linear lines radiating to and from the hilum is commonly seen. The major subjective complaint in these patients is dyspnea. Physiological testing demonstrates a restrictive defect and gas exchange is characterized by a reduction in carbon monoxide gas transfer (D_LCO) and profound hypoxemia. Since the pattern on chest X-ray and pulmonary physiology is indistinguishable from a variety of other interstitial lung diseases, a tissue diagnosis is warranted. This can usually be obtained with a transbronchial lung biopsy via flexible fiberoptic bronchoscopy or by open lung biopsy.

The patient afflicted with either Hodgkins or non-Hodgkins lymphoma is particularly challenging because of the difficulty in differentiating infectious from lymphomatous infiltrates. In a series reported by Greenman [11], 50% of their patients with lymphoma had biopsy evidence of lymphoma infiltration in resected lung specimens; Bodes [12] found that two-thirds of their patients with pulmonary complications arose in the lymphoma sub-population. An important point is that unless mediastinoscopy or thoracotomy with lung biopsy is performed, the etiology of the pulmonary lesions is frequently not diagnosed. Bronchoscopic and transthoracic needle aspiration have a low yield in lymphoma detection [13].

Lymphomatous involvement of the lung can mimic infection and drug reaction on chest X-ray with the appearance of nodules (including cavitary), localized or diffuse infiltrates, mediastinal lymphadenopathy, and pleural effusions. The lung is initially involved in 5–20% of patients with lymphoma and eventually in 20–60% [14]. Nodular sclerosing Hodgkins disease is most frequently implicated [15]. If patients have received radiotherapy to the chest and mediastinum, mediastinal and hilar lymphadenopathy is less common [16]. But, because parenchymal recurrences still occur, open lung biopsy is frequently needed for definitive diagnosis [13].

In patients with leukemia, 60–80% will develop pulmonary infiltrates at some time during the course of their disease and over 90% will have radiographic evidence of this at death [17, 18]. There are further diagnostic possibilities in the leukemic patient including infection and leukemic infiltration, direct effect of chemotherapeutic agents, alveolar hemorrhage, capillary leukostasis and forms of non-cardiac pulmonary edema related to biologic substances released by lysis of leukemic cells or produced by leukocytic proliferation.

Infection is clearly the most common cause of pulmonary infiltration in the leukemic and appears to relate directly to the degree of neutropenia [19]. Differences in etiology exist depending upon whether the patient has presented untreated or after initiation of chemotherapy. Untreated patients generally have intact lymphocyte function and more commonly present with bacterial pneumonia, leukemic infiltrates, or alveolar hemorrhage. Pneumonia is commonly seen in patients with qualitative and quantitative abnormalities of polymorphonuclear leukocytes, leukemic infiltrations in patients with very high white counts, and hemorrhage in patients with thrombocytopenia. The characteristics of the infiltrate may also be helpful. In Tenholder's series [17], those who presented with localized pulmonary infiltrates commonly were noted to have bacterial pneumonia. Less than 10% of such cases were due to opportunistic infection. Therefore, it is reasonable to empirically treat a patient presenting with leukemia and a localized process with broad spectrum antibiotics. In patients who present with diffuse infiltrative lung disease, etiologies include infection, hemorrhage, leukemic infiltration, and cardiogenic pulmonary edema. Tissue diagnosis is, therefore frequently required to establish the diagnosis. Leukemic infiltration of the lung was seen most commonly in patients with acute nonlymphocytic leukemia and chronic lymphocytic leukemia [20].

Alveolar hemorrhage has been reported in 40–60% of patients with leukemia and was frequently associated with fever and leukemic infiltrations [21, 22]. Hemoptysis occurred in less than half, but was usually accompanied by a platelet count of less than $15,000/mm^3$.

White blood cell counts of greater than $100,000/mm^3$, have been associated with extreme hypoxemia, dyspnea, and sometimes with normal chest X-rays [23]. It appears that such very high leukocyte counts cause occlusion of pulmonary capillaries and result in defects in gas exchange. In an autopsy review of 206 patients dying of leukemia [20], all patients with leukocyte counts greater than $200,000/mm^3$ had leukostasis of the pulmonary capillary bed.

Non-cardiac pulmonary edema ('capillary leak respiratory failure') has been noted in patients treated for 'blast crisis' [25]. Rapid lysis of leukemic blasts can release proteolytic enzymes that result in diffuse alveolar damage. With respiratory support, most of these patients may recover. To confirm this process (termed 'leukemic cell lysis pneumonopathy'), an open lung biopsy is required.

The mechanisms for diffuse alveolar damage in patients with leukemia are extensive. Certain infectious agents, pulmonary capillary leukostasis, lysis of blasts, production of hyperoxide radicals by polymorphonuclear leukocytes, leukemic blast thrombi, and direct effects of chemotherapeutic drugs can cause acute respiratory distress with fever, infiltration, and hypoxemia. Careful history, correlation with prior therapy, and a current laboratory database, especially including a chest X-ray, are crucial in early decision making. An early diagnosis of a treatable process may prevent acute respiratory failure, and is important to establish because of the extremely poor prognosis in patients with advanced respiratory distress undergoing ventilatory support who have sepsis, shock and/or leukopenia [26].

Pulmonary disease caused by infection

Acute infection is the most common cause of pulmonary disease in the cancer patient. However, there are several important considerations in the diagnosis of infectious infiltrates. Selected infections should be suspected based both on the type of immunological defect caused by the cancer or its treatment, and on the radiographic presentation. Epidemiologic history including travel and drug use are also helpful. The physician must analyze the pertinent data base to determine the next option for further diangosis and treatment. Figure 1 reveals a scheme used at our institution to deal with the cancer patient presenting with a new pulmonary infiltrate on chest X-ray.

Although the chest X-ray may be helpful in focusing on the etiology, most pathogens can produce most forms of roentgenographic appearance. Therefore, isolation of the pathogen by various techniques described later is often required in order to render optimal care.

Pulmonary reaction to drugs

The signs and symptoms of pulmonary disease (fever, dyspnea and infiltrates on chest X-ray) associated with drugs used for a chemotherapeutic effect are identical to those caused by infection, neoplastic infiltration of lung parenchyma, and alveolar hemorrhage. Unfortunately, there are no specific tests that implicate a specific drug. Although there are characteristic

112

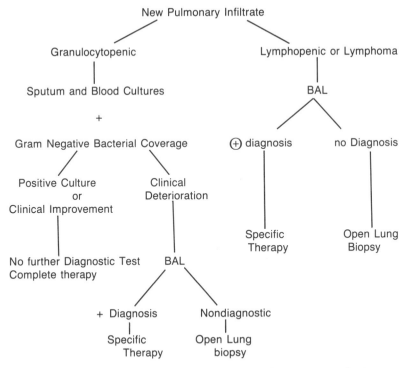

Figure 1. Evaluation of new pulmonary infiltrate. This algorithm separates the immunocompromised patient into a granulocytopenic or lymphopenic host. The former would receive gram-negative antibacterial coverage while awaiting routine cultures. If further clinical deterioration occurs, broncho-alveolar lavage (BAL) would be performed. If the patient is lymphopenic one would start with broncho-alveolar lavage; in either instance if no diagnosis is apparent after broncho-alveolar lavage then one would proceed to open lung biopsy.

histological changes seen in the lungs of patients with drug-associated pulmonary disease, the diagnosis is largely one of exclusion. One should always demonstrate the absence of neoplasm or infection and define a chronological history of cumulative drug exposure.

Adverse drug reactions can occur in patients treated for a wide variety of conditions. However, because of the toxic effects that many of the cancer chemotherapeutic agents have on cellular constituents, the lung and its delicate alveolar capillary membrane are particularly vulnerable to injury. As a consequence, the following pathophysiological pulmonary syndromes can occur: bronchospasm, interstitial fibrosis, pulmonary edema, pulmonary infiltrates with or without eosinophils, alveolar hemorrhage and acute respiratory failure due to diffuse alveolar damage.

Although the pathogenesis of drug-related tissue injury remains unknown, several mechanisms have been considered [27]. Pulmonary hypersensitivity reactions seem to be implicated particularly in methotrexate-induced pulmonary damage, whereas injury as a result of drug induced hyperoxide free radical production is thought to be the mechanism whereby bleomycin produces pulmonary toxicity [28]. Table 1 lists those cancer chemotherapeutic agents known to induce pulmonary disease [29].

The most common pulmonary reaction to cancer chemotherapeutic drugs is interstitial pneumonitis. This process is characterized histologically by thickening of the alveolar septa with chronic proliferation of interstitial lymphocytes and collagen. The 'type II' alveolar lining cells are commonly affected, producing characteristic 'round cells' bulging into the alveolar spaces and containing hyperchromatic and smudged nuclei. These were originally described with 'Busulfan Lung' [30], but have been noted with other cytotoxic drugs. Oxygen and ionizing radiation have been shown to enhance pulmonary toxicity [32, 33] providing additional evidence for the oxygen radical alveolar damage theory.

The symptoms produced by these drugs can be insidious with subacute development of non-productive cough, dyspnea, and fever. There may be the development of eosinophilia and progressive increase in alveolo-interstitial lung markings on chest X-ray. Since the alveolar capillary interface is the site of early damage, physiologic testing of respiratory gas exchange is the most sensitive way of establishing the pulmonary involvement. A decline in resting and exercise arterial pO_2, and a decrease in carbon monoxide diffusing capacity is noted and frequently precedes roentgenographic changes [34].

Gallium 67 scanning of the lungs has been effectively utilized in the early detection of drug-induced lung disease [35]. The scan reveals a patterns of diffuse alveolo-interstitial inflammation; however, it does not exclude the possibility of concomitant opportunistic infection caused by *Pneumocystis carinii* or cytomegalovirus. Frequently, histological examination of the lung

Table 1. Classification of drug-associated pulmonary injury.

Cytotoxic oxidant lung injury	Non-cytotoxic hypersensitivity reaction
Azathioprine	Bleomycin sulfate
Bleomycin sulfate	Cytosine arabinoside
Busulfan	Methotrexate
Chlorambucil	Procarbazine hydrochloride
Cyclophosphomide	
Hydroxyurea	
Melphalan	
Mitomycin	
Nitrosurea	
Procarbazine hydrocholoride	

may demonstrate the presence of both drug-induced injury and infectious processes. Unfortunately, despite cessation of chemotherapeutic drugs and intervention with corticosteroid therapy, fatalities may still occur.

Bleomycin is especially toxic to the pulmonary parenchyma and has been used in laboratory animals to study pulmonary toxicity [36]. In patients receiving this agent, about 10% develop lung injury and 1–2% go on to die [37]. Bleomycin-induced pulmonary injury is more common in patients over the age of 70 and when the cumulative dose exceeds 450 units, but reactions have occurred with doses below 200 units [38, 39]. The incidence of reactions to other cytotoxic drugs are probably less than 5% and are similar to those of bleomycin with regard to their effect on the pulmonary parenchyma [29].

Non-cytotoxic pulmonary reactions are commonly caused by methotrexate [40]. Histopathological characteristics of this type of drug include the absence of the bizarre atypia of 'type II cells', the frequency of blood eosinophilia, and the complete reversal of symptoms after cessation of therapy with the offending agent.

Rosenow has reported non-specific pneumonitis in patients with methotrexate-associated pulmonary reactions and has noted granulomas appearing in the lung tissue in one-third [41]. Symptoms frequently begin within several weeks of starting therapy and rapidly disappear when the drug is discontinued.

New pulmonary process unrelated to malignancy

During the course of disease management the cancer patient is subject to multi-organ system complications which can result in lung disease. Many of these complications are very difficult to separate from the more common pulmonary processes of infection and drug reaction previously described. However, they must always be considered by the physician because treatment and outcome may be totally different.

Left ventricular failure with resultant pulmonary edema can develop insidiously [42]. Many cancer patients receive large volumes of intravenous fluids and are in the age group where ischemic heart disease is prevalent. The findings of left ventricular failure can be subtle; manifestations may include only dyspnea and increased interstitial markings on chest X-ray. The patient's drug treatment regimen should be reviewed for agents known to produce toxicity to the myocardium (e.g., doxorubicin hydrochloride). Previous radiation treatments should be reviewed to determine whether the heart has been exposed to critical doses of ionizing radiation. If there are no contraindications, a trial of diuretics and fluid restriction is probably the easiest diagnostic maneuver.

The sedentary lifestyle common to many patients with malignancy can predispose to pulmonary thromboembolism. Patients may present with the sudden onset of tachypnea and tachycardia associated with hypoxemia. In 25% of patients with pulmonary emboli, the chest X-ray may be normal and in others there may be segmental infiltrates, regional oligemia and pleural effusions. Since the chest X-ray presentation is usually non-specific, a nuclear ventilation/perfusion lung scan and/or pulmonary angiogram should be performed to provide a definitive diagnosis [43]. The lung scan is frequently non-specific in patients with pre-existing lung disease caused either by pneumonia or chronic obstructive pulmonary disease. In such cases, unless there is a high probability scan with non-matched lobar or major subsegmental defects, the more definitive pulmonary angiogram should be performed. Since long-term anticoagulation therapy, especially in a cancer patient, is not without risk, one should firmly document the presence of pulmonary emboli in the lung or evidence of proximal deep venous phlebothrombosis in the lower extremities.

Aspiration pneumonia is a common problem in many chronically ill hospitalized patients and the cancer patient is no exception [44]. Aspiration probably contributes to the terminal event in many cancer patients who become progressively unresponsive to therapy. Whereas opportunistic organisms may infect the immuno-compromised host, these patients usually acquire bacterial superinfection with gram-negative or anaerobic microorganisms. Patients with esophageal malignancies, seizure disorders from cerebral metastasis, and obtundation from narcotics or metabolic disturbances such as hypercalcemia are particularly prone to aspiration pneumonia. If treatment is undertaken, broad spectrum, specific antibiotic treatment should be prescribed. Corticosteroids have clearly been shown to have no effect clinically on aspiration pneumonia and may actually enhance superinfection [45].

Acute non-cardiac pulmonary edema can result from many causes [46]. A recent variant of this syndrome has been described following blood transfusion [47]. It is postulated that there is a reaction between leukoagglutinating and lymphocytotoxic antibodies of the donor and the leukocytes of the recipient. It usually occurs within 4 h of the transfusion and is self-limited characterized by dyspnea, cough, fever, and hypotension. Hypoxemia and X-ray infiltrates are noted in the absence of abnormality in pulmonary capillary wedge pressures. Treatment is supportive with volume expansion, oxygen, and time. The interaction of amphotericin and leukocytes to cause leukoagglutination resulting in pulmonary infiltrates has also been described and may have a related etiology [48, 49]. In all patients who develop pulmonary parenchymal processes resulting in hypoxemia, further damage by oxygen toxicity must be avoided. High FIO_2s over 40% and high arterial pO_2s greater than 120 torr can enhance the pulmonary injury through damage by oxygen radicals [50].

Alveolar hemorrhage has been previously described in patients with hematopoetic malignancy. However, it can be seen in any patient with a depressed platelet count or alterations in clotting factors. A diagnosis is unlikely unless tissue is obtained, but it should be considered in patients with disseminated intravascular coagulation (DIC) or when severe thrombocytopenia exists (less than 15,000 platelets); treatment is supportive. When DIC exists, the cause should be eliminated if possible. Coagulation disorders and thrombocytopenia should be vigorously corrected. If the patient survives, the alveolar hemorrhage is gradually cleared by the alveolar macrophage phagocytic system.

The development of a second but unrelated neoplasm must always be considered in the cancer patient. Predisposition to a second malignancy has been postulated as secondary to a defect in immunosurveillance mechanisms and/or chemotherapeutic agents [51]. The most common second solid tumor is lung cancer in men and breast cancer in women, reflecting the situation in the normal population. The most frequent non-epithelial neoplasms in either sex are lymphomas and nonlymphocytic leukemias [52].

In patients who have received radiotherapy to the thorax for cancer management, radiation effects in the lungs can induce severe pulmonary reactions [53]. These can be either acute (especially after a large single dose), or chronic [54]. The symptoms of the acute reaction occur within several days of the radiation. Chronic radiation pneumonitis when total radiation dosage exceeds 4,000 rads, frequently occurs in the area bounded by the portals placed on the thoracic cage. The chest X-ray usually reveals sharply marginated areas of parenchymal fibrosis. Treatment of radiation pneumonitis is largely supportive. Corticosteroids have generally not been shown to have a favorable effect, but there is an isolated report of radiation pneumonitis occuring after withdrawal of prednisone during a chemotherapeutic treatment of Hodgkins disease [55].

Extrapulmonary disease – pleural effusion

Pleural effusions in the cancer patient may be due either to the neoplastic process or to a separate pleural event. The history, clinical course, and analysis of pleural fluid and/or pleural tissue helps to establish the etiology. Table 2 separates pleural effusions into transudates and exudates based on accepted criteria of pleural fluid analysis [56].

The formation of pleural fluid is a dynamic process. There is continued production and absorption of pleural fluid across the parietal and visceral pleural surface based on the Starling principle involving vascular hydrostatic pressure, tissue oncotic pressure and a capillary permeability factor [57]. When hydrostatic forces exceed net absorptive forces, a transudative effu-

Table 2. Classification of pleural fluid by biochemical analysis.

	Transudate	Exudate
Pleural fluid: plasma protein ratio	<0.5	>0.5
Pleural fluid: plasma LDH ratio	<0.6	>0.6
Absolute LDH value	<200	>200
Protein content	<3 g	>3 g
Specific gravity	<1.015	>1.015

sion is produced, as seen in congestive heart failure, hypothyroidism, or severe hypoproteinemia.

During an inflammatory state involving the pleural surface, there is increased capillary permeability or malfunction of regional lymphatic drainage preventing clearance of cellular debris and protein from within the pleural space. As a consequence, an exudative effusion develops, as seen in parapneumonic effusions, lymphoma, or metastatic mediastinal lymphadenopathy. Chemically, pleural fluid is separated into transudates and exudates based on pleural fluid serum ratio of protein LDH and absolute LDH values [56]. This separation allows one to consider the possible etiology of the effusion. Table 3 lists some of the causes of pleural fluid in the cancer patient [57].

The predominant mechanism of pleural fluid accumulation in carcinoma is tumor obstruction of the lymphatic channels draining the pleural space. An analysis of 96 patients with carcinomatous involvement of the pleura by Chernow and Sahn [58] noted no relationship between the extent of direct pleural involvement by metastatic disease and the development of a pleural effusion. However, there was a strong relationship between carcinomatous infiltration of mediastinal lymph nodes and the development of the pleural effusion. Meyers [59] demonstrated in an autopsy series of 29 patients that the pathogenesis of direct pleural metastasis was the result of direct pulmonary artery invasion and embolization of tumor to the pleural surface.

Chernow [58] found that adenocarcinoma of the lung was the most common cell type to involve the pleura whereas Meyers [59] found involvement

Table 3. Causes of transudative and exudative pleural effusions in the cancer patient.

Transudate	Exudate
Bronchial obstruction and atelectasis	Bronchial obstruction with pneumonia
Superior vena caval syndrome	Mediastinal lymph node obstruction
Hypoproteinemia	Chylothorax
Congestive heart failure	Drug reaction
Pulmonary emboli	Pulmonary emboli

in 38 % of lung cancer patients with small cell carcinoma. When bilateral pleural metastases were seen, there was almost always evidence of lymphatic spread and contralateral lung involvement.

A paramalignant effusion is defined as a pleural effusion associated with a systemic malignant process; however, not all paramalignant effusions are the result of mediastinal lymph node tumor obstructing normal flow. Transudative effusions have been seen with patients with bronchial obstruction, atelectasis, pulmonary embolism, superior vena cava syndrome, and low tissue oncotic pressure secondary to hypoproteinemia. Exudative effusions have been seen with pneumonia effusions complicated by endobronchial obstruction, chylothorax, mediastinal radiation, and drug reactions, especially to methotrexate, procarbazine and cyclophosphamide [60].

Most patients with large pleural effusions present with dyspnea on exertion and cough. However, 23 % in Chernow's series were totally asymptomatic [58]. In contrast to paramalignant effusions, patients with effusion secondary to malignant mesothelioma have a high incidence of chest pain [61]. Dyspnea and cough were the second and third most frequent symptoms with this entity.

The presence of pleural fluid can be suspected on the basis of history and careful physical examination which usually demonstrates dullness to percussion and marked decrease in breath sounds at the base of one hemithorax. Chest X-ray confirms the presence of the effusion with a classic 'meniscus sign' and contralateral mediastinal shift if the effusion is massive. A lateral decubitus film is helpful in demonstrating free fluid in preparation for diagnostic thoracentesis. Thoracentesis is always advisable, but malignant cells may not be observed because the effusion is a consequence of obstruction of lymphatic drainage. Chemical analysis of the fluid is helpful as well as additional diagnostic studies on pleural tissue. The gross appearance of pleural fluid may suggest a malignant etiology. If the fluid is bloody, it suggests the additional possibility of trauma, tuberculosis, or pulmonary infarction. A milky effusion suggests thoracic duct involvement (chylothorax) or a cholesterol effusion. A turbid fluid suggests parapneumonic etiology, and a viscous nature suggests a mesothelioma [58].

The cell count and differential of pleural fluid is rarely specific unless grossly purulent. Paramalignant effusions often demonstrate a predominance of lymphocytes, mesothelial cells and occasional eosinophils. Cytology is positive for malignant cells in only 60 % of effusions associated with malignancy. The biochemical analysis of paramalignant effusions is also variable. In Sahns's series of confirmed paramalignant effusions, 10 % were transudates and 90 % were exudates. The glucose was occasionally less than 50 mg %, 30 % had a pH less than 7.3, and 30 % had an LDH greater than 500 mg % [58]. Hyaluronic acid is increased in many cases of mesothelioma [62]. If the etiology of the pleural effusion is not clear after thoracentesis, other diagnostic procedures should be explored. Pleural biopsy increases the yield three fold and direct pleuroscopy increases the yield still further [63]. Bronchoscopy may be helpful if concomitant bronchial obstruction is suspected. In the most difficult cases, open pleural biopsy may be required for diagnosis.

The management of the patient with a malignant or paramalignant effusion may range from simple observation to pleurectomy. Obviously, the patient's general health, tumor origin and expected survival must be carefully assessed before selecting a management option. The physician must also be certain that the effusion is caused by the malignancy when management hinges on whether or not this is the case. In lung cancer, a pleural effusion usually signifies inoperability. In Decker's series, less than 5% were found to have a surgically resectable tumor if pleural fluid was present at the time of diagnosis [64].

For non-pulmonary tumors metastatic to the lung, documentation of malignant cells in pleural fluid or pleural tissue is mandatory. Patients who develop an asymptomatic paramalignant effusion after documentation of etiology may require no specific therapy unless dyspnea or pain develops. Therapeutic thoracentesis should then be performed. This rarely resolves the problem, but may allow the near terminal patient with dyspnea to better tolerate the effusion.

Systemic chemotherapy is rarely sucessful in managing malignant effusions unless the primary tumor has also responded. Tumors in which this mode of therapy can be considered include breast, small cell (lung), lymphoma, and testicular.

Radiotherapy may be attempted for radiosensitive tumors such as lymphoma or small cell carcinoma and is directed toward mediastinal lymphadenopathy. Whole lung and pleural radiation should be avoided because the adverse effects of radiation pneumonitis usually outweigh any benefit of decreasing pleural fluid formation.

Closed tube thoracostomy has been attempted but is only rarely effective without the use of intrapleural sclerotherapy. Numerous agents have been employed over the past 30 years and include nitrogen mustard, quinacrine, bleomycin, 5-florouracil, thiotepa, and talc. However, tetracycline, known for its sclerosing complications after subcutaneous infiltration, appears to be one of the best agents for pleural symphysis [65–67].

Sahn [68] showed, in an elegant experiment, that pleural symphysis is dependent on the agent's ability to cause adherence of parietal and visceral pleural rather than to any antineoplastic activity of the agent. The use of tetracycline may cause severe pain and fever, and every patient should be warned of this possibility. The discomfort can be reduced by parenteral narcotics and intrapleural lidocaine [69]. Since pleural symphysis is not without problems, it is imperative to document that the effusion is caused by a malignant process, has recurred, and relief of symptoms has occurred with fluid removal.

Control of the effusion occurs in about 85% of properly selected cases with intrapleural tetracycline. The pleural fluid pH is sometimes helpful in selecting cases for pleural symphysis [70]. Only 22% of patients with a pleural pH of less than 7.3 had successful control, whereas 83% with a pH greater than 7.3 had a good response. Therefore, if survival is expected to be several months, the patient's general condition is good and a pleural fluid pH of greater than 7.3, intrapleural instillation of tetracycline is advisable. If the patient's prognosis is poor (less than 3 months), and the pleural fluid pH is less than 7.3, repeat outpatient therapeutic thoracentesis may be preferable.

If tetracycline sclerosis is attempted, proper technique requires complete drainage of the pleural space with a closed tube thoracostomy placed in the mid axillary line and directed toward the diaphragm [66, 67]. Closed drainage should be continued until pleural fluid is minimal and the lung has re-expanded. The patient should be medicated with narcotic analgesia and the pleural space lavaged with 50 cc of saline and 15 cc of 1% lidocaine. With rotation of the patient in an attempt to coat the entire pleural surface, 20 mg/kg of body weight of tetracycline and 100 cc of saline are instilled through the pleural space for 15 min and the total pleural surface exposed to the tetracycline. The chest tube is initially clamped for 15–30 min and is then unclamped and placed under water seal with negative suction until daily tube drainage is less than 150 cc per day. The chest tube then can be safely removed and if the process was effective, reaccumulation of effusion is minimal [66, 67].

In carefully selected patients who are expected to have long-term survival, surgical pleurectomy may be attempted and is usually effective, but requires a thoracotomy [71].

Unfortunately, malignant mesothelioma, a relatively uncommon primary pleural malignancy, does not respond favorably to either modality of treatment. A few patients have survived long-term after radical de-bulking therapy of the pleural space [72]. However, controlled studies are lacking. The prognosis for this tumor is dismal and pain control is of paramount importance.

Paramalignant effusions are common, especially with lung cancer and other extrathoracic tumors metastatic to the mediastinal lymph nodes. Once the effusion is documented to be directly related to tumor, the patient enters a palliative therapeutic course directed toward relief of symptoms caused by progressive pleural fluid volume. The status of the patient's general health, biochemical characteristics of the effusion, and the expected survival, all help in selecting the preferred mode of management.

Summary of diagnostic approach

The rapidity of onset of a new pulmonary process must be assessed in order to appropriately guide diagnostic studies. In general, one starts by discontinuing all unnecessary drugs and proceeds with a standard laboratory data base of complete blood count, SMA-12, and chest X-ray. The following additional non-invasive and invasive procedures may be helpful.

Non-invasive diagnostic procedures

Analysis of sputum
If a parenchymal process is discovered, an expectorated sputum should be examined if available. A direct gram stain should be obtained with the knowledge that many leukopenic cancer patients will probably not have polymorphonuclear leukocytes in their sputum. To be sure the material is sputum, it should contain either fewer than 10 squamous cells per low power field and/or more than 25 alveolar macrophages or leukocytes per low power field. A negative gram stain does not exclude a bacterial pneumonia, but a predominance of one or more organisms seen on direct smear may be helpful in guiding initial antibiotic therapy. Alternative decisions can be made based on subsequent culture and other smears for acid fast organisms, fungi, and legionella. Unfortunately, the yield from direct sputum examination is low.

Serology
IgG antibodies against mycoplasma, fungi, legionella, cytomegalovirus, and toxoplasmosis can be demonstrated in the blood of infected subjects. Acute infection should be suspected if a four-fold rise in titer can be demonstrated. A titer of ≥1:256 for legionella is strongly suggestive of active legionella infection [73]. With the exception of fungal immunodiffusion tests which identify preciptin bands, these serological tests usually require paired acute and convalescent sera 2 weeks apart. This is obviously unlikely to be of help in a rapidly deteriorating patient. However, some fungal serologies can be processed early but false positive and false negative results are common. Detection of cryptococcal polysaccharide antigen in blood or CSF is strongly suggestive of crytococcosis [74].

Body fluids
Culture of the blood, pleural fluid, CSF, urine and other body cavities is relevant in screening for a source of infection. Newer blood culturing techniques have increased the yield of fungi and mycobacteria isolated from blood [75].

Invasive diagnostic procedures

A number of reports have established the transtracheal needle aspiration as a means of providing uncontaminated secretions from the lower tracheo-bronchial tree [76]. It has been helpful in identifying anaerobic organisms, but these are infrequent infections in the cancer patient. The bleeding complications that can occur in cancer patients who are frequently thrombocytopenic and the low yield of the procedure has made many clinicians abandon this procedure in favor of obtaining secretions from deeper within the lung.

Bronchoscopy
The flexible fiberoptic bronchoscope with special double lumen catheter enables one to obtain semi-quantitative cultures of bacteria from the diseased pulmonary segment [77]. In patients who have radiographic evidence of diffuse disease and are not thrombocytopenic or seriously hypoxemic, the technique of a transbronchial lung biopsy through the fiberoptic scope provides lung tissue for histological review, culture, and special stains for microorganisms [78]. The technique of broncho-alveolar lavage with 200 cc of normal saline, lavaged via the flexible fiberoptic bronchoscope into a segmental bronchus, has provided additional data when the lavage pellet is reviewed with special stains and cultures [79]. Due to oral cavity contamination by *Candida* species and bacteria, bronchial lavage has limited value. However, broncho-alveolar lavage smears and brushings are helpful in identifying fungi, other than *Candida* species, *Pneumocystis carinii,* mycobacteria and *Legionella* species [80]. At our institution, the Infectious Disease, Pulmonary and Microbiology services have established a team protocol for handling broncho-alveolar lavage and open lung biopsy specimens. Within 3 h, one can obtain a gram stain, AFB smear, rapid silver methenamine for pneumocystis and fungi, and a direct fluorescent antibody (DFA) for *Legionella* [81] (see Table 4).

Table 4. Evaluation of protocol for broncho-alveolar lavage and open lung biopsy specimens

Smear	Culture	Histopathology
Gram stain	Routine bacteria	Routine hematoxylin
acid fast stain	Anaerobic bacteria	and eosin
GMS[a] stain –	Mycobacteria	GMS[a]
pneumocytsis/fungi	Fungi	Acid fast
DFA[b] stain –	*Legionella*	
Legionella	Viruses	

[a] GMS = gomori methenamine silver.
[b] DFA = direct fluorescent antibody.

Percutaneous transthoracic aspiration

Percutaneous transthoracic needle aspiration is associated with two major disadvantages. Firstly, diagnosis of infection is difficult because sample size is small. Secondly, there are risks of pneumothorax and serious intrapulmonary hemorrhage [82]. Since many centers report higher complication rates in sick cancer patients, open lung biopsy may be preferred for this patient population.

Thoracoscopy with pleural biopsy

The use of the thoracoscope within the pleural space has recently been advocated to obtain parenchymal lung tissue [83]. Although yields of interpretable tissue may be as high as 64% there are riks of pneumothorax and uncontrollable hemorrhage.

Open lung biopsy

Open lung biopsy often provides the most definitive and safest diagnostic procedure. In critically ill subjects, the airway can be controlled and complications related to hemorrhage or airleak may be effectively managed. At our institution, rapidly deteriorating patients receive open lung biopsy using the protocol outlined above (Table 4) to process the lung tissue. If the patient's course is less acute, we prefer initial studies employing flexible fiberoptic bronchoalveolar lavage and transbronchial lung biopsy. Both procedures can be performed safely in most patients by monitoring oxygenation, cardiac rhythm, and alveolar ventilation. Open lung biopsy can also be safely performed in a patient with thrombocytopenia by infusion of platelets shortly before the procedure.

Rapid assessment of the cancer patient with a new pulmonary process is critical. Because the differential diagnosis of a new pulmonary process in the cancer patient is so extensive, a systematic approach toward diagnosis is imperative. The sound judgement and the diagnostic resources of the oncology-pulmonary-infectious disease team has been very important in establishing a rapid diagnosis of the pulmonary process and initiating appropriate treatment.

References

1. Singer C, Armstrong D, Rosen PP, Walzer PD, Yu B. 1979. Diffuse pulmonary infiltrates in the immunosuppressed patient: Prospective study of 80 cases. Am J Med 66:110–120.
2. Williams DM, Krick JA, Remington JS. 1976. Pulmonary infection in the compromised host. Am Rev Respir Dis 114:359–394, 593–627.
3. Burrows B, Earle RH. 1969. Course and prognosis of Chronic obstructive lung disease. NEJM 280:397–404.
4. Demeter SL, Ahmad M, Tomaskefski JF. 1979. Drug induced pulmonary disease – I. Pat-
5. terns of response; II. Categories of drugs; III. Agents used to treat neoplasms or alter the

immune system including a brief review of radiation therapy. Cleve Clin Q 46:89–99, 101–112, 113–124.

6. Samter M, Beers RF. 1968. Intolerances to aspirin: clinical studies in consideration of its pathogenesis. Ann Intern Med 68:975–983.

7. Nash G: 1982. Pathologic features of the lung in the immunocopromised host. Hum Pathol 13:841–858.

8. Holmes EC, Ramming KP, Eilber FR. 1977. Surgical management of pulmonary metastasis. Sem. Oncol 4:65–69.

9. Kessel L. 1959. Spontaneous disappearance of bilateral pulmonary metastases. Report of a case of adenocarcinoma of kidney after nephrectomy. JAMA 169:1737–1739.

10. McCormack DM et al. 1978. Pulmonary resection in metastatic carcinoma. Chest 73:163–166.

11. Janower ML, Blennerhassett JB. 1971. Lymphangitic spread of metastatic carcinoma of the lung. Diagn Radiol 101:267–273.

12. Greenman RL, Goodall PT, D. 1975. Lung biopsy in immunocompromised hosts. Am J Med 59:488–496.

13. Bode FR, Pare JA, Fraser RG. 1974. Pulmonary diseases in the compromised host: A review of clinical and roentgenographic manifestations in patients with impaires host defense mechanisms. Medicine (Baltimore) 53:255–293.

14. Harlan JM, Fennessy JJ, Gross NJ. 1974. Bronchial brush biopsy in Hodgkin's disease. Chest 66:136–138.

15. Filly R, Blank N, Castellino RA. 1976. Radiographic distributions of intrathoracic disease in previously untreated patients with Hodgkin's disease and non-Hodgkin's lymphoma. Radiology 120:277–281.

16. Whitcomb ME, Schwarz MI, Keller AR, Flannery EP, Blom J. 1972. Hodgkin's disease of the lung. Am Rev Respir Dis 106:79–85.

17. Costello P, Mauch P. 1979. Radiographic features of recurrent intrathoracic Hodgkin's disease following radiation therapy. Am J Roentgenol 133:201–206.

18. Tenholder MF, hooper RG. 1980. Pulmonary infiltrates in leukemia. Chest 78:468–473.

19. Bodey GP, Powell RD Jr, Hersh EM, Yeterian A, Freireich EJ. 1966. Pulmonary complications of acute leukemia. Cancer 19:781–793.

20. Balducci L, Halbrook JC, Chappan SW, Vance RB, Thigpen JT, Morrison FS. 1983. Acute leukemia and infections: perspectives from a general hospital. Am j Hematol 15:57–63.

21. Klatte EC, Yardley J, Smith EB, Rohn R, Campbell JA. 1963. The pulmonary manifestation and complications of leukemia. Am J Toentgentol 89:598–609.

22. Wardman AG, Milligan DW, Child JA, Delamore IW, Cooke NJ. 1984. Pulmonary infiltrates in adult acute leukemia: empirical treatment and survival related to the extent of pulmonary radiological disease. Thorax 39:568–571.

23. Tenholder MF, Hooper RG. 1980. Pulmonary hemorhage in the immunocompromised host: An Elusive reality (Abstract). Am Rev Respir Dis 121 (Suppl):198.

24. Vernant JP, Brun B, Mannoni P, Dreyfus B. 1979. Respiratory disease of hyperleukocytic granulocytic leukemias. Cancer 44:264–268.

25. McKee LC Jr, Collins RD. 1974. Intravascular leukocyte thrombi and aggregates as a cause of morbidity and mortality in leukemia. Medicina (Baltimore) 53:463–478.

26. Tryka AF, Godleski JJ, Fanta CH. 1982. Leukemic cell lysis pneumonopathy: A complication of treated myeloblastic leukemia. Cancer 50:2763–1770.

27. Fowler AA, Hamman RF, Zerbe GO, Benson KN, Hyers TM. 1985. Prognosis after onset of adult repiratory distress syndrome. Am Rev Respir Dis 132:472–478.

28. Sostman Matthay RA, Putman CE. 1977. Cytotoxic drug induced lung disease. Am J Med 62:608–615.

29. Ginsberg SJ, Comis RL. 1982. The pulmonary toxicity of antineoplastic agents. Sem Oncol 9:34–51.

30. Rosenow EC III. 1980. Chemotherapeutic drug induced pulmonary disease. Sem Respir Med 2:89–96.
31. Heard BE, Cooke RA. 1968. Busulphan lung. Thorax 23:187–193.
32. Green MR. 1977. Pulmonary toxicity of antineoplastic agents. West J Med 127:292–298.
33. Tyrka AF, Skornik WA, Godleski JJ, Brain JD. 1982. Potentiation of bleomycin induced lung disease by exposure to 70% oxygen: Morphologic assessment. Am Rev Respir Dis 126:1074–1079.
34. Einhorn L, Krause M, Hornback N, Furnas B. 1976. Enhanced pulmonary toxicity with bleomycin and radiotherapy in oat cell lung cancer. Cancer 37:2414–2416.
35. Manning DM, Straimlan CV, Turbiner EH. 1980. Early detection of husulfan lung: Report of a case. Clin nucl Med 5:412–414.
36. MacMahon H, Bekerman C. 1978. The diagnostic significance of gallium lung uptake in patients with normal chest radiographs. Radiology 127:189–193.
37. Bedrossian CWM, Greenberg SD, Yawn DH, O'Neal RM. 1977. Experimentally induced bleomycin sulfate pulmonary toxicity. Arch Pathol Lab Med 101:248–254.
38. Blum RH. 1974. An overview of bleomycin pulmonary toxicity. In: New drug Seminar on Bleomycin. National Cancer Institute, Bethesda, Maryland, pp 151–162.
39. Holoye PY, Luna MA, MacKay B, Bedrossian CWM. 1978. Bleomcyin hypersentitivity pnemonitis. Ann Intern Med 88:47–49.
40. Perez-Guerra F, Harkleroad LE, Walsh RE, Costanzi JJ. 1972. Acute bleomycin lung. Am Rev Respir Dis 106:909–913.
41. Sostman HD, Matthay RA, Putman CE, Walker Smith GJ. 1976. Methotrexate induced pneumonitis. Medicine (Baltimore) 55:371–388.
42. Rosenow EC III, Unni KK. 1983. Drug Induced granulomas. Lung Biol Health Dis 20:469–484.
43. Rosenow EC III, Harrison CE Jr. 1970. Congestive heart faillure masquerading as primary pulmonary disease. Chest 58:28–36.
44. Moser KM, Fedullo PF. 1983. Venous Thromboembolism: Three simple decisions. Chest 83:117–121, 256–260.
45. Barlett J, Gorbach S. 1975. The triple threat of aspiration pneumonia. Chest 68:562–566.
46. Downs J. 1974. An Evaluation of steroid therapy and aspiration pneumonitis. Anesthesiology 40:129–135.
47. Fowler AA, Hamman RF, Good JT, Benson KM, Baird M, Eberle DJ, Petty Tl, Hyers TM. 1983. Adult respiratory distress syndrome: risk with commonpre-dispositions. Ann Intern Med 98:593–597.
48. Popovsky MA, Abel MD, Moore SB: 1983. Transfusion related acute lung injury associated with passive transfer of anti-leukocyte antibodies. Am Rev Respir. Dis 128:185–189.
49. Wright DG, Robichaud KJ, Pizzo PA, Deisseroth AB. 1981. Lethal pulmonary reactions associated with the combined use of amphotericin B and leukocyte transfusions. N Engl J Med 304, 20:1185–1189.
50. Boxer LA, Ingraham LM, Allen J, Oseas RS, Baehner RL. 1981. Amphotericin B promotes leukocyte aggregation of nylon-wool-fiber-treated polymorphonuclear leukocytes. Blood 58, 3:518–23.
51. Clark JM, Lambertsen CJ. 1971. Pulmonary oxygen toxicity – A Review. Pharmacol Rev 23:37–133.
52. Reiner RR. 1982. Risk of a second malignancy related to the use of cytotoxic chemotherapy. CA 32:286–292.
53. Penn I. 1976. Second malignant neoplasms associated with immunosuppressive medications. Cancer 37:1024–1032.
54. Gross NJ. 1977. Pulmonary effects of radiation therapy. Ann Intern Med 86:81–92.
55. Smith JC. 1963. Radiation pneumonitis. Am Rev Respir. Dis 87:647–655.
56. Castellino RA, Glastein E, Turbow MM, Rosenberg S, Kaplan HS. 1974. Latent radiation injury of lungs or heart activated by steroid withdrawal. Ann Intern Med 80:593–588.

126

57. Light RW, MacGregor I, Luchsinger PC, Ball WC. Pleural effusions: The diagnostic separation of transudate and exudates. Ann Intern Med 77:507–513.
58. Black LF. 1972. The pleural space and pleural fluid. Mayo Clin Proc 47:491–506.
59. Chernow B, Sahn SA. 1977. Carcinomatous involvement of the pleura: An analysis of 96 patients. Am J Med 63:695–702.
60. Meyer PC. 1966. Metastatic carcinoma of the pleura. Thorax 21:437–443.
61. Rosenow EC III. 1980. Miscellaneous drug induced pulmonary disease. Semin Respir Med 2:76–88.
62. Oels H, Harrison E, Carr D. 1971. Diffuse malignant mesothelioma of the pleural: A review of 37 cases. Chest 60:565–570.
63. Kwel WS, Veldhuizen RW, Goldring RD, Mullink H, Stam J, Donner R, Boon ME. 1982. Histologic distinction between malignant mesothelioma, benign pleural lesion and carcinomatous metastasis. Virchows Arch (Pathol Anat) 397:287–299.
64. Boutin C, Viallat JR, Cargnino P, Farisse P. 1981. Thoracoscopy in malignant pleural effusion. Am REV Respir Dis 124:588–592.
65. Decker DA, Dines PE Payne WS: 1978. The significance of a cytologically negative pleural effusion in bronchogenic carcinoma. Chest 74:640–642.
66. Sahn SA, Good JT JR, Potts DE. 1979. The pH of sclerosing agents: A determinate of pleural symphysis. Chest 76:198–200.
67. Wallach HW. 1975. Intrapleural tetracycline for malignant effusions. Chest 68:510–512.
68. Zaloznik AJ, Oswald SG, Langin M. 1983. Intrapleural tetracycline inmalignant pleural effusions: A randomized study. Cancer 51:752–755.
69. Sahn SA, Good JT Jr. 1981. The effect of common sclerosing agents on the rabbit pleural space. Am Rev Respir Dis 124:65–67.
70. Wallach HW. 1978. Intrapleural therapy with tetracycline and lidocaine for malignant pleural effusions. Chest 73:246.
71. Good JTJr, Taryle DA, Sahn SA. 1978. Pleural fluid pH in malignant effusions: Pathophysiologic and prognostic implications. Chest 74:338.
72. Martini N, Bains MS, Beattie EJ Jr. 1975. Indications for pleurectomy in malignant effusions. Cancer 35:734–738.
73. Butchart EG, Ashcroft, T, Barnsley WC: 1981. The role of surgery in diffuse malignant mesothelioma of the pleura. Sem. Oncol 8:321–328.
74. Beaty HN, Miller AA, Broome CV, Goings S, Phillips CA: 1978. Legionnaires' disease in Vermont. JAMA. 240, 2:127–131.
75. Fisher ED, Armstrong D. 1977. Cryptococcal interstitial pneumonitis: Value of antigen determination. NEJM 297:1440–1444.
76. Pierce PF, DeYoung DR, Roberts GD. 1983. Mycobacteremia and the new blood culture systems. Ann Intern Med 99:780–789.
77. Ries K, Levision Me, Kaye D. 1974. Transtracheal aspiration in pulmonary infection. Arch Intern Med 133:453–458.
78. Wimberly N, Faling LJ, Bartlett JG. 1979. A fiberoptic bronchoscopy technique to obtain uncomtaminated lower airway secretions for bacterial culture. Am Rev Respir Dis 119:337–343.
79. Stover DE, Zaman MB, Hajdu SI, Lange M, Gold J, Armstrong D. 1984. Bronchoalveolar lavage in the diagnosis of diffuse pulmonary infiltrates in the immunosuppressed host. Ann Intern Med 101:1–7.
80. Kelly J, Landis JN, Davis GS, Trainer TD, Jakob GJ, Green GM. 1978. Diagnosis of pneumonia due to pneumocystis by subsegmental pulmpnary lavage via the fibreroptic bronchoscope. Chest 74:24–28.
81. Rankin JA. 1985. Bronchoalveolar lavage for research purposes in the immunocompromised host. Chest 88:319–320.
82. Landis JN, Jaciow D. Personal communication.

83. Zavala DC, Schoell JE. 1981. Ultrathin needle aspiration of the lung in infectious and malignant disease. Am Rev Respir Dis 123:125–131.

84. Dijkman JH, van der Meer JWM, Bakken W, Wever AMJ, van der Brock PJ. 1982. RTranspleural lung biopsy by the transthoracic route in patients with diffuse interstitial pulmonary disease. Chest 82:76–83.

9. The use of psychotropic medications in the treatment of cancer

DANIEL J. FRIEDENSON

'Yes, life was there and now it is going, going and I cannot stop it. Yes. Why deceive myself? Isn't it obvious to everyone but me that I'm dying, and that it's only a question of weeks, days... it may happen this moment. There was light and now there is darkness. I was here and now I'm going there! Where?'. A chill came over him, his breathing ceased, and he felt only the throbbing of his heart.

'When I am not, what will there be? There will be nothing. Then where shall I be when I am no more? Can this be dying? No, I don't want to!'.

From: *The Death of Ivan Ilych*, Leo Tolstoy.

Introduction

This chapter will focus on the use of psychotropic medication to treat depression, anxiety, and acute confusion and agitation. Psychotropic medications are almost certainly underused in patients with cancer. A frequent lack of appreciation of the patient's level of emotional distress, particularly depression [1], coupled with a certain therapeutic nihilism, may account for this lack of vigor in an area where the physician actually stands a good chance of helping the patient. Psychotropic drug use in seriously ill patients requires special care. The presence of significant cardiac, pulmonary, hepatic, renal, gastrointestinal, or endocrinologic disease may create specific pharmacologic dilemmas. The discussion of psychotropic drug use in cancer patients which follows is, by necessity, selective. Any reader wishing a more comprehensive discussion of these specific situations is referred to several excellent reviews [2–5].

Higby, DJ (ed), Issues in Supportive Care of Cancer Patients. ISBN 0-89838-816-3.
© 1986, Martinus Nijhoff Publishers, Boston. Printed in the Netherlands.

Depression

Depression is probably the most common psychiatric illness seen in medical outpatients and inpatients. Various studies have suggested that 15–40% of medical outpatients are significantly depressed. One would expect a similar prevalence of depression in patients with malignancy. One careful study [6] done with patients hospitalized for chemotherapy of solid tumors, lymphoma, and leukemia found approximately 25% of patients either moderately or severely depressed. While some investigators [7] have found significant depression in 37% of randomly selected radiotherapy patients, another recent survey [8] of nearly 200 patients in home-based and hospital-based hospice programs reveals that only 6% of patients were taking antidepressant medication. In one university center [9], less than 2% of annual cancer admissions were referred for psychiatric evaluation. Of these, 56% were suffering depression. These representative figures certainly suggest that depression in cancer patients is underrecognized and undertreated. In an attempt to account for this disparity, one is forced to examine attitudinal factors. It seems only natural that an individual faced with pain, increasing physical debility, loss of function, altered body image, separation from loved ones, forced dependency, unpleasant diagnostic and therapeutic maneuvers, and a bleak or uncertain future might be discouraged. Statements such as, 'Of course he's depressed' or 'I'd be down too, if I were in her shoes' reflect this view. Unfortunately, this superficial logic may dull our appreciation of the persistence or severity of a patient's depression and dissuade us from pursuing vigorous therapy. In fact, depression which has begun in response to agreeably disappointing, sad, or fearsome events may develop an independent 'life of its own', which further debilitates the patient and robs him of what pleasures and tranquility he might otherwise experience in his last weeks or months. Although antidepressant medication cannot alter 'depressogenic' events, it can successfully treat the signs and symptoms of depression. More harm has probably been done by undertreating depressed patients than by overtreating them.

Indications for treatment

In an otherwise healthy individual, depressive illness is characterized by some or all of the following signs and symptoms: loss of appetite; sleep disturbance (most often early morning awakening) not caused by physical discomfort; decreased energy; loss of interest in previously pleasurable activities (anhedonia); decreased libido; feelings of guilt, worthlessness, hopeless, and helplessness; crying; suicidal ideation. In a classically depressed patient, this syndrome is most severe in the morning, although this is not always the case. The presence of vegetative signs (changes in appetite, sleep, energy level, libido) of sufficient duration (2 or 3 weeks) is usually indication for treatment in a healthy individual. Since patients undergoing treatment for cancer may have some or all of the classically 'vegetative' signs as a result of physical illness or side effects of its treatment, these signs may be less reliably diagnostic, although still suggestive. Special emphasis should, therefore, be placed on evaluating the psychological symptoms of depression. It has been noted that patients with cancer, although frequently discouraged, do have moments of optimism and cheerfulness and seldom display impaired self-esteem, preoccupation with feelings of guilt and worthlessness, or relentless dysphoria [6]. Presence of these non-somatic depressive symptoms for more than 2 or 3 weeks is strong indication for treatment.

Pharmacology of antidepressants

Ten heterocyclic antidepressants are in common use at this time (see Table 1). Several more will be introduced within the next 2 years. Most antide-pressant medications are weakly basic compounds which are well-absorbed in the small intestine and then strongly bound to serum proteins (the small unbound fraction of medication is the pharmacologically active form). They are metabolized to inactive compounds principally by the hepatic cyto-chrome P-450 system prior to renal excretion. The mechanism of action of these medications is not entirely clear. Originally, it was thought that they exerted their antidepressant effect via blockade of neurotransmitter (cate-cholamine and indolamine) reuptake (and destruction), thus effectively increasing the supply of neurotransmitter. Recent evidence [10] has sug-gested that alteration of central post-synaptic receptor sensitivity may ac-count for their antidepressant effect.

Side effects of antidepressant medication

The principal side effects of antidepressant medication are cardiac, antichol-inergic, autonomic-hypothalamic, and central nervous system.

Some clinicians approach prescribing antidepressants with undue wari-ness about their potential cardiac toxicity. Most of the data about the car-diotoxic effects of antidepressant medication stems from observations of patients who have overdosed (parenthetically, numerous observers have noted that suicide attempts are infrequent in cancer patients). Except when used in overdose attempts or in patients with a history of ventricular irri-tability or dysrhythmia, these medications are quite safe. Their main cardiac

Table 1. Heterocuclic antidepressants.

	Sedative potency	Anti-cholinergic potency	Orthostatic hypotensive potency	Cardiac arrhythmogenic potential	Starting dose (mg/day)	Target dose (mg/day)	Dose range (mg/day)
Older heterocyclis							
1. Tertiary amines							
Doxepin (Sinequan, Adapin)	High	Moderate	Moderate	Yes	50	200	75–300
Amitriptyline (Elavil)	High	Very high	Moderate	Yes	50	150	75–300
Imipramine (Tofranil)	Moderate	Moderate	High	Yes	50	200	75–300
Trimipramine (Surmontil)	High	Moderate	? Moderate	Yes	50	150	75–300
2. Secondary amines							
Protriptyline (Vivactyl)	Low	High	Low	Yes	15	30	15–60
Nortriptyline (Aventyl, Pamelor)	Moderate	Moderate	Low	Yes	25–50	100	40–140
Desipramine (Norpramin, Pertofrane)	Low	Low	Low	Yes	50	150	75–300
Newer heterocyclis							
Amoxopine (Asendin)	Moderate	Low	? Low	Yes	50	200	75–400
Maprotiline (Ludiomil)	Moderate	Low	? Low	Yes	50	150	75–225
Trazodone (Desyrel)	Moderate	Very low	Moderate	Yes	50	150	50–600

* Give early in day to avoid interference with sleep.

Note: Elderly patients or those with cerebral impairment require lower (1/2 to 1/3) starting dose and target dose.

effects are antivagal and quinidine-like. The increased heart rate occasionally seen at low doses is an antivagal side effect. At therapeutic doses, atrioventricular and intraventricular conduction times are sometimes increased, resulting in a prolonged Q-T interval. Orthostatic hypotension (probably related to the antidepressants' ability to relax vascular smooth muscle) can be problematic, particularly in the elderly, who are more susceptible to variations in blood pressure and are more likely to experience injury if they do fall. All patients starting antidepressant therapy should be warned to take several extra seconds when arising from a supine or sitting position, and to be alert to lightheadedness in situations such as a hot shower, where blood pressure often drops anyway.

Antidepressants exhibit varying degrees of anticholinergic activity, manifest principally as dry mouth, blurred vision, delayed micturition, and constipation. Dry mouth is most often a curiosity or minor annoyance. Occasionally, it can become a major problem, exacerbating dental or periodontal disease. Chewing gums or candy used to stimulate salivation can have the same untoward effects. Sugar-free gums and candies are preferred. Low doses of bethanecol or neostigmine have proven effective in stimulating salivation in some refractory cases of xerostomia. Blurred vision (caused by interference with normal accommodation mechanisms) is seldom a limiting factor in antidepressant use. This side effect, if it occurs, usually abates within days. Antidepressants have been reported to precipitate acute worsening of narrow angle glaucoma. The physician must be cautious to use an appropriate topical agent before instituting antidepressant therapy. Anticholinergic inhibition of bladder contraction can cause urinary retention in patients with prostatic hypertrophy or those in whom urethral patency is compromised. In a patient without significant outflow obstruction, bethanecol is useful in treating delayed micturition or urinary retention. However, one should take caution in using cholinergic agents when significant outflow obstruction is present. Some urologists fear this may lead to damage to, or even rupture of, the bladder wall. Constipation can usually be treated by using stool softeners or water-retaining laxatives. In patients with precarious gastrointestinal motility (e.g., post-op abdominal surgery patients or those with partial GI obstruction), fecal impaction or adynamic ileus may occur.

Appetite stimulation, weight gain, and sweating are hypothalamic-autonomic side effects seen with antidepressant use. Amitriptyline is most likely to stimulate appetite, while imipramine has been most strongly associated with unwanted (and poorly understood) axillary and truncal sweating.

At therapeutic doses, antidepressant medication can cause a fine intention tremor, which rarely is problematic. Sedation is not an uncommon side effect during the first week of antidepressant therapy. Since many depressed patients suffer sleep disturbance, this side effect can be utilized by giving antidepressants in a single dose shortly before bedtime whenever possible. Some individuals report vivid dreaming and, occasionally, nightmares while taking antidepressants. This response is somewhat idiosyncratic, and reassurance (in the case of vivid dreaming) or switching to an alternate antidepressant (in the case of nightmares) is usually effective in addressing these problems. Antidepressants theoretically lower seizure threshold, although this is rarely a clinical problem. Maprotoline (Ludiomil), however, has been noted to cause an increased frequency of seizures in doses greater than 225 mg per day. This potential difficulty is not a contraindication to using antidepressants in an individual with a history of seizure disorder. Rather, the informed physician should take appropriate measures to assure that anticonvulsant blood levels are in therapeutic range. Elderly patients, those with cerebral pathology (e.g., stroke, tumor, etc.) or those taking other sedating medications may experience confusion or agitation when given antidepressants. These side effects seem related to the central anticholinergic effect of antidepressants. Presence of other signs of peripheral cholinergic blockade (dry mucous membranes, sluggishly responsive pupils, flushing, increased body temperature) can help support a diagnosis of 'atropine psychosis'. The syndrome is treated by withholding the antidepressant and repeatedly reorienting and reassuring the patient. There is usually significant resolution over 24–36 h. When pharmacologic intervention is necessary for this 'atropine psychosis', physostigmine 1–4 mg i.m. or i.v. q2h p.r.n. has proven useful. Low dose, high potency antipsychotic medication (e.g., Haldol 0.5 mg p.o. b.i.d. or t.i.d.) may help. In fact, this latter intervention is seldom necessary. After the syndrome has cleared, a less anticholinergic antidepressant (Table 1) can be instituted.

Significant drug interaction

The use of heterocyclic antidepressants in combination with other potentially sedating drugs, such as antihistamines, narcotic analgesics, barbiturates, non-barbiturate sedative hypnotics, or benzodiazepines may result in unexpected sedation. Likewise, antihistamines or antiparkinsonian drugs in combination with antidepressants may enhance the likelihood of an anticholinergic delirium developing. Antispasmodics, sympathomimetics, and antiparkinsonian medications may delay gastric emptying and thus promote acid breakdown of antidepressants in the stomach. Methylphenidate, barbiturates, diphenylhydantoin, primidone, and oral anticoagulants may inhibit hepatic hydroxylating enzymes and may thus lead to increased blood levels of antidepressants. Antipsychotics and heterocyclic antidepressants utilize the same hepatic cytochrome P-450 enzyme system and this may interfere with each other's metabolism when used simultaneously.

Effects of organ impairment

Any impairment in gastric emptying will enhance acid breakdown of anti-depressants and thus effectively decrease the amount of medication which reaches the systemic circulation. Since the cytochrome P-450 system is present in the diseased as well as the healthy liver, hepatic disease does not always cause impaired antidepressant metabolism. Standard initial doses, but gentler dose graduation are advised. Since heterocyclic antidepressants are for the most part metabolized and eliminated by the liver, they can be used in normal doses in patients with renal failure.

Choice of agent

Although no antidepressant has been demonstrated to be statistically more effective than any other, a given individual may respond better to one agent than another. Careful history-gathering is, therefore, of primary importance. A candidate for antidepressant treatment should be asked about any previous periods of depression and treatments with antidepressant medication. Much time has been wasted in failed medication trials because these simple questions were never asked. Prior positive response to a specific antidepressant in either the patient or a family member is the single most important piece of history a clinician can uncover. In general, presuming a patient's tolerance for side effects has not changed dramatically since a prior course of treatment, one should always prescribe an antidepressant which has worked successfully before. If the patient has no prior personal or family history of successful treatment for depression, one's choice of antidepressant medication is determined by knowledge of differential side effect profiles (Table 1). In general, among the standard tricyclic agents, demethylated derivatives (desipramine, nortriptyline) have lower side effect (anticholinergic, cardiac, CNS, hypothalamic-autonomic) profiles than their parent compounds (imipramine, amitriptyline). Amitriptyline, doxepin, and maprotilime are the most sedating antidepressants. This side effect may be desirable in cases where sleep disturbance is a particularly prominent symptom. Conversely, in cases where minimal sedation is wished, desipramine, or protriptyline, may be preferable. Amitriptyline, imipramine, and doxepin are the most anticholinergic antidepressants. Desipramine is the least anticholinergic of the standard tricyclics and may be particularly useful in cases where urinary retention or adynamic ileus is feared. Nortriptyline, and desipramine, are the least 'hypotensogenic' of the antidepressants. Although all antidepressants have cardiac arrythmogenic potential, the actual incidence of cardiac arrythmias *is* low. Desipramine, and maprotoline, are reasonable choices when one wishes to minimize risk of cardiac arrythmia.

Dosages of antidepressants

Target doses and dose ranges for the heterocyclic antidepressants are listed in Table 1. One aims to reach target dose by the end of the second week of treatment. Of note is that the elderly are more susceptible to side effects (sedation, confusion, hypotension, and parasympathetic blockade) and should, therefore, be started at lower doses, with smaller and more gradual dose increments. In general, one expects the starting and target doses for an elderly patient to be one-half to one-third of the normal adult target dose. Most antidepressants should be given in a single dose shortly before bedtime. In some patients, desipramine is mildly 'alerting' and should be given during the day. Peak-related antidepressant side effects can be managed by using divided doses.

Response

Emergence from depression occurs in a stepwise fashion. Sleep is often improved immediately, owing to the sedative side effects of most antidepressants. In general, some beginning signs of response to medication are seen by the middle to end of the second week of treatment. Signs (total hours of sleep, level of animation, food consumption) often improve before symptoms (anxiety, sadness, self-deprecation, etc.). Once target dose is reached, it should be kept constant as long as the patient is improving. If the patient plateaus at a sub-optimal response, the dose of antidepressant may then be increased incrementally. If the patient returns to his euthymic (pre-depression) state, he should then be maintained on antidepressant medication for 3–5 months, after which the dose should be tapered by 20–25% per week (some patients may report a surge of vivid dreaming if antidepressants are withdrawn too rapidly). If signs of depression re-emerge, the dose should be increased immediately.

Anxiety

Anxiety is characterized by motor tension, autonomic hyperactivity, apprehensive expectation, and vigilance and scanning. The ideal antianxiety medication should dampen or remove these symptoms without causing undue sedation. Benzodiazepines clearly perform this function better than any other class of medication (e.g., neuroleptics, barbiturates, antihistaminic sedations, narcotics) used to treat anxiety. This discussion of drug treatment of anxiety will, therefore, focus on benzodiazepines. These effective medications are prescribed for 15% of adult Americans every year. In one recent year, two billion benzodiazepine tablets and capsules were prescribed in the United States. In one survey at New York Hospital, 44% of medical inpatients and 64% of surgical inpatients had benzodiazepines available to them. Given the fearsome nature of cancer, one would expect the prevalence of significant anxiety and benzodiazepine usage in cancer patients to match or exceed that in the general population. It is therefore somewhat surprising that one large multicenter study [11] reported that 25% of oncology patients received an antianxiety medication, while a more recent survey of data derived from the National Hospice Study [8] revealed that 16% of cancer patients in the last weeks of life were prescribed benzodiazepines.

Metabolism of benzodiazepines

As a rule, benzodiazepines are well-absorbed when given orally (Tranxene must undergo gastric acid hydrolysis prior to absorption), are lipophylic, and bind strongly to serum protein. The longer-acting agents (Valium, Librium, and Tranxene) are more lipophylic and thus more rapidly and widely distributed. When taken orally, they have a more rapid onset than agents with shorter half-lives (Ativan, Serax, Xanax, etc.), but their lipophylicity may result in unpredictable serum levels when they are given parenterally, due to deposition in subcutaneous adipose tissue [12]. Although all benzodiazepines are metabolized in the liver, Serax, Ativan, and Restoril have the simplest metabolism, involving only conjugation with glucuronic acid. The other benzodiazepines have several active metabolites and depend on the hepatic mixed-function oxidase system for their metabolism. Thus, Serax, Ativan, and Restoril are preferred antianxiety medications in patients with impaired hepatic function. All benzodiazepines are excreted principally via the kidney. Thus, appropriate downward titration of dose should be made in patients with impaired renal function.

Side effects of benzodiazepines

Unlike the heterocyclic antidepressants and the antipsychotic medications, the benzodiazepines are essentially free of autonomic, anticholinergic, and extrapyramidal side effects. Their principal potential aide effect, sedation, can usually be avoided by careful titration of dosage. They share very few significant drug-drug interactions, but may have a synergistic sedating effect when used in combination with other potentially sedating medications, such as narcotics, antihistamines, heterocyclic antidepressants, and barbiturates. Medication orders should always be written so as to avoid giving antianxiety medication to a patient who is already drowsy.

Dosing strategies

The benzodiazepines currently in use in the United States are listed in Table 2. The dichotomy between those used to induce sleep and those used to treat anxiety is somewhat artificial, reflecting drug marketing (and subsequent research) strategies rather than significant pharmacological differences. The 'antianxiety' benzodiazepines are usually given in divided doses (three or four times per day), although the longer-acting agents (Valium, Librium, Tranxene) can be given once daily after steady state conditions are reached. As can be seen in Table 2, benzodiazepines marketed as anxiolytics all come in 'small, medium and large' pill or capsule doses, while those marketed as hypnotics (Dalmane, Restoril, Halcion) come in 'small and large' sizes. Except for Serax, Librium, Centrax, Dalmane, and Restoril, all

Table 2. Comparison of benzodiazepines.

Drug	Onset[a]	Normal half-life (hours)[b]	Active meta-bolites	Pill/capsule dose (mg)	Total daily dose (mg) Adult	Elderly
Anxiolytics						
Alprazolam (Xanax)	I	6–20[b]	Yes	0.25, 0.5, 1.0	0.75–3	0.75–1.5
Oxazepam (Serax)	S	5–15	No	10, 15, 30	10–60	10–30
Lorazepam (Ativan)	I	10–20	No	0.5, 1, 2	1–6	0.5–3
Diazepam (Valium)	R	20–100[b]	Yes	2, 5, 10	5–30	2–10
Chlordiazepoxide	I	5–30[b]	Yes	10, 25, 50	10–100	5–30
Prazepam (Centrax)	S	36–200[b]	Yes	5, 10, 20	20–60	10–15
Clorazepate dipotassium (Tranxene)	R	36–200[b]	Yes	3.75, 7.5, 15	15–30	7.5–15
Hypnotics						
Flurazepam (Dalmane)	R	40–250[b]	Yes	15, 30	30	15
Triazolam (Halcion)	I	5	No	0.25, 0.5	0.5	0.25
Temazepam (Restoril)	S	8–22	No	15, 30	30	15

[a] R = rapid; I = intermediate; S = slow.
[b] Half-life may be prolonged in cases of significant hepatic illness.

benzodiazepines are available as scored tablets. In general, it is reasonable to initiate treatment with a specific anxiolytic using the smallest dose size three or four times per day, and thereafter titrating the dose upward every 2 or 3 days as needed. When longer-acting agents (Valium, Librium, Tranxene, Centrax) are used, dose increments should be smaller and less frequent (every 4 to 5 days) to avoid oversedation secondary to drug accumulation. As in the case of antidepressants, the elderly should receive one-third to one-half the normal adult dosage, and subsequent dosage increments should be equally cautious.

Caution

Restlessness due to medication side effects (as with terbutaline) or an acute confusional state (see following section) may mimic 'normal' anxiety. In these cases, a change in medication or correction of any correctible imbalances or intoxications are the respective treatments of choice. Likewise, antianxiety medication is an ineffective substitute for vigorous analgesia in a patient whose painful restlessness has been mistaken for anxiety.

Agitation and confusion secondary to organic brain syndrome

The functional psychoses (manic-depressive illness, schizophrenia, major depressive disorder with psychotic symptoms) are relatively rare in medical inpatients. In the huge majority of cases, acute agitation or psychosis (i.e., delusional thinking with or without hallucinations) in hospitalized medical patients in general, and cancer patients in particular, is caused by structural or chemical derangement or cerebral functioning.

Organic brain syndrome is defined as a collection of psychological and behavioral signs or symptoms resulting from diffuse impairment of brain tissue functioning from any cause. Historically, the term 'delirium' (synonyms: metabolic encephalopathy, acute confusional psychosis, organic psychosis) has been used to describe the relatively acute, *usually* reversible organic brain syndrome in which the 'lesion' is chemical rather than structural. Dementia describes those organic brain conditions which are gradual in onset (months to years), usually progressive, and in which gross pathology (e.g., atrophy, space-occupying lesions) is usually evident. Although both delirium and dementia can be seen in cancer patients, delirium is the more common cause of acute agitation and psychosis and will be the principal focus of discussion here. Although only the most dramatic cases reach formal psychiatric attention, the prevalence of organic brain syndrome in a general hospital is high. The prevalence of delirium has been conservatively

Cognitive Capacity Screening Examination

Examiner _____ Date _____

Instructions: Check items answered correctly. Write incorrect or unusual answers in space provided. If necessary, urge patient once to complete task.

Introduction to patient: "I would like to ask you a few questions. Some you will find very easy and others may be very hard. Just do your best."

Addressograph Plate

1) What day of the week is this? _____

2) What month? _____

3) What day of month? _____

4) What year? _____

5) What place is this? _____

6) Repeat the number 8 7 2. _____

7) Say them backwards. _____

8) Repeat these numbers 6 3 7 1. _____

9) Listen to these numbers 6 9 4. Count 1 through 10 out loud, then repeat 6 9 4. (Help if needed. Then use number 5 7 3.) _____

10) Listen to these numbers 8 1 4 3. Count 1 through 10 out loud, then repeat 8 1 4 3. _____

11) Beginning with Sunday, say the days of the week backwards. _____

16) The opposite of large is _____

17) The opposite of hard is _____

18) An orange and a banana are both fruits. Red and blue are both _____

19) A penny and a dime are both _____

20) What were those words I asked you to remember? (HAT) _____

21) (CAR) _____

22) (TREE) _____

23) (TWENTY-SIX) _____

24) Take away 7 from 100, then take away 7 from what is left and keep going: 100 - 7 is _____

25) Minus 7 _____

26) Minus 7 (Write down answers; check correct subtraction of 7) _____

12) 9 + 3 is _____

13) Add 6 (to the previous answer or "to 12"). _____

14) Take away 5 ("from 18'').
   Repeat these words after me and remember them,
   I will ask for them later: HAT, CAR, TREE, TWENTY-SIX.

15) The opposite of fast is slow. The opposite of up is _____

27) Minus 7 _____

28) Minus 7 _____

29) Minus 7 _____

30) Minus 7 _____

TOTAL CORRECT (maximum score = 30) _____

Patient's occupation (previous, if not employed) _____ Education _____ Age _____
Estimated intelligence (based on education, occupation, and history, not on test score):

Below average, Average, Above average _____

Patient was: Cooperative _____ Uncooperative _____ Depressed _____ Lethargic _____ Other _____

Medical diagnosis: _____
IF PATIENT'S SCORE IS LESS THAN 20, THE EXISTENCE OF DIMINISHED COGNITIVE CAPACITY IS PRESENT.
THEREFORE, AN ORGANIC MENTAL SYNDROME SHOULD BE SUSPECTED AND THE FOLLOWING
INFORMATION OBTAINED.

Temp. _____ BUN _____ Endocrine dysfunction? _____ T_3, T_4, Ca, P, etc.

B.P. _____ Glu _____ History of previous psychiatric difficulty _____

Hct _____ Po_2 _____

Na _____ Pco_2 _____ Drugs: _____ Steriods? L-Dopa? Amphetamines? Tranquilizers? Digitalis?

K _____

Cl _____ Focal neurological signs: _____

CO_2 _____

EEG _____ DIAGNOSIS: _____

ECG _____

Figure 1. Cognitive capacity screening examination.

estimated to be 5% [13]. The diagnosis is often missed. In one study [9], significant organic brain syndrome was undetected by the referring physician in 26 of 100 consecutive cancer patients referred for psychiatric evaluation. A central feature of delirium is global impairment of wakefulness and alertness, often punctuated by moments of clarity. The patient may oscillate between mild drowsiness and extreme arousal. Any or all of the following functions may be affected to varying degrees.

1. *Orientation.* Orientation to time is most fragile, followed by orientation to place and person. Many medical inpatients will mistake the day of the week by 1 day and the day of the month by 1 or 2 days. More serious error should raise suspicions of organicity.
2. *Memory.* Recent memory is more fragile than long-term memory, although both may be affected.
3. *Attention.* This may be reduced or fluctuate, with easy distractibility.
4. *Insight.* The ability to appreciate one's situation (e.g., that one is ill, the nature and gravity of the illness, the nature of the treatment) may be subtly or dramatically impaired.
5. *Thought content and process.* Disorganization of thought, racing thoughts, blocking, perseveration, and confabulation may all be seen. Delusions, when present, are usually transient, unsystematized, and persecutory.
6. *Perception.* Illusions (misinterpretations of actual sensory stimuli) or hallucinations (sensory perceptions without an actual stimulus) may occur. Non-auditory hallucinations (i.e., visual, tactile, olfactory, or gustatory) should raise strong suspicions about organicity.

Of note is that although global (i.e., involving many or all areas of psychological functioning), the deficits exhibited by delirious patients may be extremely subtle and evident only after very careful observation. Patients with organic brain disorders may be aware of and attempt to hide their deficits. In hospitalized medical patients, any psychological or behavioral phenomenon of relatively acute onset, which waxes and wanes and worsens at night ('sundowning'), suggests delirium. Several simple questionnaires have been developed to screen for organic brain syndromes. One, the Cognitive Capacity Screening Examination, is relatively easy to use and is reproduced on pages 140-141 (Figure 1) [14].

Table 3 contains a selective listing of causes of organic brain syndrome in patients with cancer. Of special interest to those involved in oncology are the neuropsychiatric side effects of chemotherapeutic agents. Mechlorethamine, hexamethylamine, dacarbazine, intrathecal methotrexate, vincristine, mithramicin, L-Asparaginase, procarbazine, and Mitotane have all been associated with acute organic brain disorder [15]. One recent excellent review [16] of psychiatric side effects of corticosteroid therapy reached the following conclusions.

Table 3. Causes of organic brain syndrome in patients with cancer.

A. *Metabolic*
1. Electrolyte – hyper or hyponatremia, hyper or hypokalemia, hypomagnesemia, hypercalcemia (secondary to bony metastases), acidosis or alkalosis
2. Hepatic failure
3. Renal failure
4. Hypoglycemia or ketoacidosis

B. *Endocrine*
1. Cushing's syndrome
2. Inappropriate antidiuretic hormone secretion
3. Excess parathormone secretion

C. *Ventilation – perfusion deficits*
1. Cardiac pathology
2. Pulmonary pathology
3. Shock-hypovolemia

D. *Sepsis and fever*

E. *Direct or indirect effect of malignancy on brain function*
1. Primary brain tumors
2. Cerebral metastases
3. Remote effects of cancer on the CNS [18]

F. *Medications*
1. Sympathomimetics
2. Anticholinergics
3. Digoxin (Foxglove Frenzy)
4. Antiarrythmics – lidocaine, Pronestyl, Inderal
5. Anticonvulsants
6. Antihypertensives (e.g., Aldomet)
7. L-dopa
8. Cimetidine
9. Barbiturates and non-barbiturate sedative hypnotics
10. Benzodiazepines – particularly longer-acting agents (Valium, Tranxene, Librium, Dalmane)
11. Antidepressants
12. Steroids and ACTH
13. Narcotics
14. Antineoplastics [15]

1. Euphoria, depression, and psychosis are the common psychiatric manifestations of corticosteroid therapy.
2. Dosage of corticosteroid correlates with risk of developing a mental disturbance, but not wish its time of onset, duration, severity, or type.
3. Females are more prone than males to these psychiatric side effects.
4. Corticosteroid-induced mental disturbances are usually reversible with dose reduction or discontinuation of corticosteroid medication.

Of note is that in one study of a group of consecutively admitted cancer patients [17], chemotherapy was the major variable associated with cognitive impairment. Lastly, it should be emphasized that systemic cancer has been associated with acute organic brain syndrome in the absence of any evidence of cerebral metastases [18]. The cause of this phenomenon is poorly understood.

Diagnostic strategies

A meticulous chart review is of the utmost importance. Nurses' notes are particularly valuable in documenting the onset and fluctuation of unusual behavior or confusion. In general, one searches for evidence of fever, metabolic imbalance, oxygenation-perfusion deficit, or the introduction of a new medication, and tries to demonstrate a temporal correlation between these changes and the observed change in mental status. If no recent laboratory studies are available, a CBC, serum electrolytes, and SMA-12 or other similar screening panel should be obtained. If a 'culprit' has been identified, one tries to correct the appropriate imbalance or remove or reduce the dosage of the offending medication. If neither metabolic imbalance nor medication side effect can be implicated, one should rule out direct cerebral involvement with tumor or infection. In such cases, a CAT scan and/or lumbar puncture may be indicated.

Non-pharmacologic treatment

By definition, individuals with organic brain syndrome are having difficulty remembering, concentrating, maintaining orientation, and assessing environmental cues. Accordingly, every effort should be made to minimize the need for new learning and to make the patient's environment as familiar and predictable as possible. Staff members should introduce themselves each time they re-enter the patient's room. The patient should have any planned tests or procedures explained several times before they are actually performed. A calendar (preferably the kind with one date per page) and a clock should be placed within easy view to aid in orientation. A familiar item from home, placed near the patient's bed, can also aid in making the environment more familiar (and, therefore, less frightening).

The use of antipsychotic medication

In cases of significant agitation or frank psychosis, antipsychotic medications can be of great benefit. They are often effective in relieving confusion, agitation, delusional thinking, and hallucinations while those causal factors which can be corrected are being corrected. While these medications do not differ in their antipsychotic effectiveness, they do differ in their milligram potency and side effect profiles. In the relatively low doses used to treat acute organic brain syndrome, sedation, hypotension, and extrapyramidal syndromes are the principal significant side effects. Acute dystonia (most often affecting the muscles of the neck, jaw, tongue, and extraocular eye muscles), akathisia (uncontrollable motor restlessness), and Parkinsonism are the extrapyramidal side effects most likely to occur during short-term antipsychotic medication use. If extrapyramidal side effects occur, a standard antiparkinsonian agent, such as Cogentin 0.5 mg p.o. t.i.d., usually ameliorates the symptom. In general, the agents with lower milligram potency (Thorazine, Mellaril, Serentil) cause more sedation and hypotension, while the more potent agents (Haldol, Prolixin, Navane) are more likely to produce extrapyramidal side effects. At the relatively low doses used to treat agitation and/or psychosis accompanying organic brain disorders, the high-potency antipsychotics are well-tolerated and are the prefer-

Table 4. Commonly used antipsychotic agents.

Non-proprietary name	Trade name	Total daily dosage (mg) (give as divided dose)	Side effects		
			Sedative effects	Extra-pyramidal effects	Hypotensive effects
Tricyclics					
1. Phenothiazines					
Chlorpromazine ** (oral)	Thorazine	30–100	***	**	*** (i.m.)
Thioridazine	Mellaril	30–100	***	*	**
Fluphenazine	Prolixin	1–3	*	***	*
Perphenazine	Trilafon	4–12	**	***	*
Trifluoperazine	Stelazine	2–6	*	***	*
2. Thioxanthenes					
Thiothixene	Navane	2–8	*–**	**	*
Other heterocyclic compounds					
Haloperidol	Haldol	1–4	*	***	*

*   Mild
**   Moderate
***   Severe

146

red agents. Table 4 is a selective listing of antipsychotic medications and dose ranges used in treating patients with organic brain syndrome.

Special mention must be made of treatment approaches to corticosteroid-induced psychoses. When possible, dosages should be reduced or corticosteroids stopped entirely. When this is not feasible, adjunctive antipsychotic medication may be used. With patients known to have had psychotic reactions to corticosteroid treatment, prophylactic treatment with lithium carbonate prior to a course of steroid-containing chemotherapy may be useful in preventing drug-induced affective psychoses. One interesting study [19] in patients receiving ACTH for treatment of multiple sclerosis has found lithium carbonate to be of statistically significant prophylactic value in preventing corticotropin-induced psychoses. A thorough review of the pharmacology of lithium is beyond the scope of this chapter. When its use is being considered, a psychiatric consultation should be obtained.

Acknowledgement

I thank Joan Panetta for her valued assistance in preparing this manuscript.

References

1. Derogatis LR, Abeloff MD, McBeth DD. 1976. Cancer patients and their physicians in the perception of psychological symptoms. Psychosomatics 17:197–201.
2. Risch SC, Groom GP, Janowsky DS. 1981. Interfaces of psychopharmacology and cardiology – Part one. J Clin Psych 42:23–34.
3. *Ibid.* 1981. Interfaces of psychopharmacology and cardiology – Part two. J Clin Psych 42:42–59.
4. Hershey SC, Hales RE. 1984. Psychopharmacologic approach to the medically ill patient. Psych Clin North Am 7:803–816.
5. Siris SG, Rifkin A. 1981. The problem of psychopharmacology in the medically ill. Psych Clin North Am 4:379–390.
6. Plumb MM, Holland J. 1977. Comparative studies of psychological function in patients with advanced cancer; I. Self-reported depressive symptoms. Psychosom Med 39:264–276.
7. Peck A. 1972. Emotional reactions to having cancer. J Roentgenol Rad Ther Nucl Med 114:591–599.
8. Goldberg RJ, Mor V. 1905. A survey of psychotropic use in terminal cancer patients. Psychosomatics 26:746–748.
9. Levine PM, Silberfarb PM, Lipowski ZJ. 1978. Mental disorders in cancer patients: A study of 100 psychiatric referrals. Cancer 42:1385–1391.
10. Charney DS, Menkes DB, Heninger GR. 1981. Receptor sensitivity and the mechanism of action of antidepressant treatment. Arch Gen Psych 38:1160–1180.
11. Derogatis LR, Feldstein M, Morrow G, Schmale A, Schmitt M, Gates C, Morawski B, Holland J, Penman D, Melisaratos N, Enclow AJ, Adler LM. 1979. A survey of psychotropic drug prescriptions in an oncology population. Cancer 44:1919–1929.

12. Shader RI, Greenblatt DJ. 1977. Clinical implications of benzodiazepine pharmacokinetics. Am J Psych 134:652–656.
13. Lipowski Z. 1967. Delirium, clouding of consciousness, and confusion. J Nerv Ment Dis 145:134–162.
14. Jacobs JW, Bernhard MR, Delgado A, Strain JJ. 1977. Screening for organic mental syndromes in the medically ill. Ann Intern Med 86:40–46.
15. Peterson LG, Popkin Mk. 1980. Neuropsychiatric effects of chemotherapeutic agents for cancer. Psychosomatics 21:141–153.
16. Ling MHM, Perry PJ, tsuang MT. 1981. Side effects of corticosteroid therapy: psychiatric aspects. Arch Gen Psych 38:471–477.
17. Silberfarb PM, Philibert D, Levine PM. 1980. Psychological aspects of neoplastic disease: II. Affective and cognitive effects of chemotherapy in cancer patients. Am J Psych 137:597–601.
18. Shapiro WR. 1976. Remote effects of neoplasm on the central nervous system: Encephalopathy. In: Advances in Neurology, Vol. 15 Thompson RA, Green JR (eds), pp 101–117.
19. Falk WE, Mahnke MW, Poskanzer DC. 1979. Lithium prophylaxis of corticotropin-induced psychosis. JAMA 241:1011–1012.

10. Psychological sequelae in the cured cancer patient

DAVID F. CELLA

Introduction

Because cancer can strike at any age, it has been called 'the most feared disease of the 20th century' [1]. The popular press often uses the word cancer as a metaphor to depict the malignant spread of anything from pollution to crime and terrorism. The 'cancer = death' equation was reflected in the pre-1970 psychosocial oncology literature, which almost exclusively emphasized the dying process and coping with terminal illness. Not until recently has close attention been paid to the psychological impact of cancer upon the millions of people who are alive and healthy long after treatment ends.

Attention to the problems of the surviving cancer patient has paralleled the progress of medical science in the treatment of cancer. In the early 1900s, surgery was the only treatment, so cure was possible only when the lesion was detected early and completely excised. The introduction of radiation therapy in the 1930s, and the addition of chemotherapy in the 1950s have dramatically improved the prognosis for many types of cancer. At present, a projected 40% (50% if one excludes death from other causes) of cancer patients diagnosed this year will still be alive in 5 years [2, 3]. Many of them will be off treatment, and may go on to live out their full life span. However, the 'disease-free' former cancer patient must have life-long vigilance toward symptoms of relapse. Cancer in these circumstances is therefore better defined as a chronic life threatening illness than as a fatal disease. Thus, today's 'cured' cancer patient faces the same tasks as those suffering from any serious chronic illness. The National Cancer Institute has identified two general tasks which the cancer patient must confront: coping with illness and its complications, such as pain or paralysis; and coping with life as it is altered by illness [4]. This chapter is concerned with the second of these tasks.

Medical advances in cancer treatment have left behind a legacy: that most successfully treated cancer patients must face a new spectrum of prob-

Higby, DJ (ed), Issues in Supportive Care of Cancer Patients. ISBN 0-89838-816-3.
© *1986, Martinus Nijhoff Publishers, Boston. Printed in the Netherlands.*

lems that are related to the late (physiological) effects of treatment. D'Angio and Ross [5] have stated: 'The normal physiology of virtually every organ or structure of the body can be impaired more or less by radiation therapy, chemotherapy and their combinations' (p. 45). Consequently, whereas multimodal therapies have had dramatic positive effects on the survival rates of some cancers, they have also increased the risks of morbidity and mortality in the post-5-year period. These include heightened risk of second malignancies, increased risk of carditis, pericarditis, pneumonia and other kinds of organ failure, susceptibility to infection, and sterility which may be permanent. Because of this, the study of late, or delayed psychological impact of cancer and its treatment is necessary.

Historically, the conceptualization of diagnosis [6], the experience of illness itself [7], and the initiation of treatment [8, 9] have been seen as stressors which disrupt homeostatic functioning in patients with life-threatening illness. At present, the majority of studies of cancer adjustment address adaptation to diagnosis and treatment. Another clinical event associated with psychological disruption is disease recurrence, frequently responded to with elevated depression and anxiety, because the patient is confronted with the failure of treatment [10, 11]. Increases in anxiety and depression are also expected at cessation of a successful course of treatment, when the patient faces separation from the security of the therapy milieu and re-entry into the 'realm of the healthy' [12-14]. Studies have shown that measures of global adaptational capability [15], coping adequacy [16], ego strength [17], and level of distress [18], differentiate poor from good adjustment during these periods. That is, some have succeeded in predicting which patients will adjust poorly during stressful treatment and survival periods. But most of these studies carry the limitations of retrospective methodology.

In an era of successful cancer treatments, the next logical step in psychosocial adaptation research is the investigation of long-term sequelae. In a recent comprehensive review article, the understanding of the long-term impact of cancer is identified as one of the key questions which remains unanswered in psychosocial oncology [19]. Of course, information in this area is essential to the development of systematic supportive care and intervention programs for cancer survivors.

Cancer patients in treatment are constantly confronted with the realization that they are different. They must make adjustments to account for the unique stressors of untimely disease and debilitating treatment. Cancer survivors must cope with chronic uncertainty about bodies that have to some extent failed them, and with frequent reminders of their past treatment ordeal. While this chapter will focus on the variety of difficulties and needs in this group, it will also support the conclusion that most survivors cope extraordinarily well with survivorship. To date, fruitful investigations have been those which have identified salient issues and patterns of adjustment to successful cancer treatment; rather than those which have looked for outright psychiatric disturbance or serious maladjustment. This chapter will review the literature on the late psychological and psychosexual effects of successful treatment. After presenting a conceptual background, the review will be divided into studies which have addressed the early survival period, known as the period of re-entry; and studies of sequelae which have been reported more than 6 months after treatment completion.

Background literature

Early Work

As early as the 1950s, Sutherland and others had clinically identified a heightened incidence of post-treatment anxiety and depression in successfully treated cancer patients [22–24]. Their work was primarily with breast and colon cancer patients. Systematic investigation of these observations pinpointed examples of anxiety about recurrence (including hypochondriacal concerns), development of dependent personality features, and increases in obsessive-compulsive and paranoid reactions, as well as general family strife [23]. Sutherland postulated that a cancer patient's pattern of adaptation, defined as 'a system of beliefs and behavior designed in order to bring the individual's physical and emotional needs in harmony with the demands of the environment', is threatened by cancer. With the homeostasis of the organism threatened, the patient is then subjected to loss of self-esteem and anxiety secondary to the subjective isolation of being a cancer patient. Bard and Sutherland [24] followed 20 breast cancer patients prospectively, from the pre-operative period to recovery. From their findings, they formulated three phases of adaptation to mastectomy (and cancer treatment in general): (1) anticipatory phase, where the patient speculates with fear and uncertainty about the damage to self and disruption of previous levels of adaptation; (2) operative phase, where the actual injury (crisis) occurs; and (3) reparative phase, where the patient attempts to re-establish the previous level of adaptation by a variety of techniques.

Holland [1] has outlined eight common psychiatric syndromes seen in cancer patients. Six of them hold some relevance to patients in the reparative phase of adaptation. They are: (1) acute stress reactions such as reactive anxiety and depression, including prolonged or delayed reactions to survival and cure; (2) major psychiatric disorders with onset during or after treatment; (3) anxiety disorders such as conditioned nausea or vomiting, phobias, and panic reactions; (4) somatoform disorders such as hypochondriasis; (5) psychosexual disorders resulting from the illness or treatment; and (6) personality disorders which can complicate and interfere with posttreatment adjustment. 'Quality of life' after treatment depends to a great extent upon the patient's prior level of emotional adjustment and the presence of emotionally supportive persons in the environment [1, 20].

Cancer as a crisis

The concepts of crisis and stress management are relevant inasmuch as adaptation to cancer survival entails some measure of protracted distress. Illness itself is a stressor which can lead to organism distress [25, 26]. Crisis theory would predict that individuals with cancer cope through a gradual integration of this life-threatening crisis [20, 21]. The term 'gradual' is intentionally vague, raising the possibility that the adjustment period could extend well into the disease free survival period.

Lindemann [27] pioneered the study of the stress response after bereavement and loss, and this concept has more recently been applied to cancer patients [26, 28]. Cancer patients during treatment have been found to use alternating combinations of intrusive and avoidant thinking styles [28]. This pattern of coping seems similar to, though less dramatic than, that found in stress response clinic outpatients.

Caplan [25] has presented a model for understanding the stress response behavior of cancer patients. His focal construct is 'mastery', defined as behavior which reduces the physiological and psychological manifestations of emotional arousal during and shortly after the stressful event; and which mobilizes one's internal and external resources, thereby developing new capabilities for changing the environment or one's relation to the environment. Presumably, these changes will either reduce the threat of the event (i.e., cancer) or replace losses (i.e., health and certainty about the future) with new sources of satisfaction.

Caplan posits four interdigitating phases of mastery in the face of stress: the first is escape or avoidant behavior which enables the individual to tolerate the intensity of the stress; the second involves acquisition behavior in which the individual attempts to change unfortunate circumstances and their aftermath. These first two phases parallel the periods of diagnosis and treatment. The third and fourth phases are more relevant to survival. Phase three entails intrapsychic behavior which defends against intrapsychic emotional arousal. Denial or avoidance of anxiety, hostility, depression, and grief are the most common mechanisms. The fourth and final phase involves synthetic intrapsychic behavior which integrates the stressful experience (diagnosis and treatment) and its sequelae (chronic uncertainties) by internal readjustment.

These 'internal readjustments' made during the reparative phase of cancer adjustment have not been well-studied, and the difficulty in measuring the defenses and inner thoughts postulated by Caplan makes his particular model untestable. However, there are some interesting recent findings which point to promising avenues of study in this regard. For example, Taylor [29, 30] has proposed that cancer patients are compelled to adjust to the threat of illness and recurrence by deceiving themselves into believing they have control. The need for this illusion is centered around three themes: the search for meaning, the effort to regain mastery (control), and the effort to maintain or enhance self-esteem. According to Taylor, this illusion provides a buffer against distress about having cancer.

Concurrent with this is the implicit assumption found in many articles on coping with cancer: that somehow the right mental outlook and the right coping style will not only contribute to subjective well-being but may even fight the disease or prevent recurrence. Based upon this reasoning, we would expect cancer survivors to have 'come to terms' with why they became ill, and to have re-organized their outlook and their lives to regain control over their bodies and health. While this may be true in a fair number of survivors, it does not seem true in the majority. In studies of cancer patients [31] and bereaved parents and spouses after sudden death of a loved one [32, 33], half of the participants never searched for the meaning in the experience. The 'why me?' question simply never got asked. And what was most interesting was that in both of these studies, using entirely different samples and measures, there was far less distress in the group that never searched for meaning than in the group which had searched. Although searching for and finding a comforting explanation may be better than searching and not finding, ironically, it seems better not to have searched at all. Another implication of these findings, in an era which promotes self-responsibility and a positive mental attitude toward disease is that people may be experiencing pressure to confront and change their outlook and behavior even though this has no proven medical efficacy and may heighten psychological vulnerability.

Following the general idea of crisis theory, that individuals resolve crises within 6 to 8 weeks [34], Lewis, Gottesman, and Gutstein [35] studied 35 cancer patients over a 28-week period after surgery. They found this notion of rapid crisis resolution not applicable to their cancer sample. Measuring anxiety, helplessness, depression, self-esteem, and general level of crisis, five variables considered to be basic indicators of crisis, they found that scores were still rising eight weeks after surgery, regardless of its outcome. At 28 weeks, however, scores did begin to decline. The results suggested either the inapplicability of a straightforward crisis model for cancer patients or the need for modification of the time frame. In another study [36], both cancer and surgery groups scored higher than healthy women on the Halpern Crisis Scale. However, the cancer sample appeared significantly more helpless than the surgery patients. Discriminant function analysis resulted in 73–82% accuracy of placement into the three groups, suggesting that cancer surgery and surgery for non-malignant conditions may represent separate types of crisis. The increase in helplessness in the cancer sample was evidence for a different, perhaps more depressive, reaction in that group. This provides indirect evidence for cancer adaptation as a process which is distinct from and more prolonged than adaptation to general medical illness and surgery. Prolonged crisis has also been documented in studies of bereaved samples [32, 33].

Re-entry: the early survival period

Chronologically, the first event associated with adaptation to cancer survival is the return to premorbid lifestyle immediately after treatment ends. The process of re-entry of the treated cancer patient into society's mainstream and the return to premorbid lifestyle has been referred to as the 'Lazarus Syndrome'. This analogy to the biblical character who returned from the dead comes from the many accounts of patients being perceived by significant others as either dead or dying during the treatment period [37, 38]. The termination of treatment and re-entry into 'normal' life can be seen as a stressor in itself, characterized by a letdown of the struggle against death and the challenge of return to normalcy [12, 13, 38].

Case reports of post-treatment disruption of socialization, financial security, vocational development, and sexual functioning are abundant in the literature [38–41]. Some of the intruding factors in this disruption include lowered self-esteem [39, 42] increased anxiety [39, 43] death-related concerns and uncertainty about the future [14, 40, 43–45] and disruption of defense mechanisms [5, 46, 47]. Cohen and Wellisch [40] describe the surviving patient and family as thrown into a state of chronic catastrophe – a psychosocial 'limbo' – where current relationships and future plans are constantly off balance because of disease uncertainty. Their observations were based upon patients *recently* completing treatment, so it is unclear how long this persists.

There have been some systematic empirical studies of cancer patients in the 6-month period following diagnosis and treatment. Weisman and Worden [48] studied 120 cancer patients over a 100-day period following diagnosis. They found that as treatment progressed, patients viewed their cancer more as a threat to their life plans (career, marriage, family) than as a direct threat to their life. They identified a 100-day post-diagnosis period, called the 'existential plight', in which fears of abandonment, loneliness, loss of control, pain, panic and the unknown were high. These concerns lessened most quickly in the Hodgkin's disease ($N = 18$) and breast cancer ($N = 37$) patients, as compared to lung ($N = 23$), colon ($N = 23$), and melanoma ($N = 19$) patients. This observation of different peak distress points for dif-

ferent cancer sites signifies the importance of studying disease sites separate-
ly rather than under the general rubric of cancer.

In a comprehensive but short-term follow-up of 308 treated breast, lung
and melanoma patients [49], interviews were conducted at four points in
time over a 6-month period (point of diagnosis, point of hospital discharge,
3 months after discharge and 6 months after discharge). Assessment was
done by semi-structured interview and a short battery of psychological tests.
In this sample, the main problem at diagnosis was worry about disease,
whereas by the time of hospital discharge it had shifted to difficulties with
negative affects such as depression, anxiety and anger. At 3- and 6-month
follow-up, problems were more widely distributed (and reduced in intensity)
across the following areas: physical discomfort, concern about treatment,
mobility, finances, family/marital problems, social problems, worry about
disease, negative affects, and disturbed body image.

Many investigators have attempted to identify patients at high risk for
maladaptation to cancer treatment and survival. Two general approaches to
this have been the study of defenses or coping style in good versus poor
adjusters, and empirical efforts to correlate pre-treatment psychological test
scores with post-treatment adjustment. The first approach has, in almost
every investigation, identified the ubiquitous and highly adaptive nature of
'denial' during the treatment and early post-treatment periods [16, 46, 50].
However, the functional adaptability of denial lessens as remission extends
and some investigators have identified an actual increase in psychological
distress and disturbance in the off-treatment period, presumably due to the
lifting of denial and exposure to the denied affects of depression, anxiety,
and hostility [45, 47]. Some data are inconsistent with this, including accounts that psychological distress tends to drop over time [5, 85], and that
longer survival times have also been associated with patients who have been
able to maintain smooth relationships with family and friends [58, 59].

It is important to separate biological outcome from psychological outcome in cancer survival. Given the connection some [52–54] have claimed
between a 'fighting spirit', and survival, and between 'stoicism' and disease
progression [51, 103], it may be that expression of distress, or at least of
feelings, has survival value. This association has not been by any means
clearly established [55, 56], nor has a consistent definition of 'fighting spirit', self-expression, or stoicism emerged which can be tested across disease
sites. This area is most important and promising for future research.

Fighting spirit notwithstanding, many prominent investigators of cancer
survival [15, 48, 57] have concluded that optimal coping with successful
post cancer treatment is not blind (unconscious) denial, but a conscious
suppression of negative emotions only after they are felt. This does not
imply stoicism, but rather a deliberate effort not to allow oneself to be
defeated by the experience and its memory. The distress and uncertainty are
acknowledged, but not centralized in the personality organization.

The second general approach to studying post-treatment psychosocial difficulty is the attempt to identify patients at high risk for psychological distress in the post-treatment period with the use of pre-treatment parameters. Using examiner ratings of post-treatment distress in patients six months off treatment, Weisman and Worden [60] were able to account for 40–60% of the variance of psychological distress with knowledge of disease stage and prognosis. That is, medically sicker patients were significantly more distressed 6 months off treatment. Other studies have found little [49] or no [61] relationship between disease or treatment severity and post-treatment distress, while some studies [62, 63] have found pre-treatment anxiety and depression to be better predictors than disease or treatment severity, of post-treatment distress in patients less than 1 year off treatment.

In a comprehensive study [18], 133 cancer patients were followed over 6 months. Pre-treatment MMPI scale scores (especially on the 'neurotic triad' of hypochondriasis, depression, and hysteria) accounted for 41% of the overall variance of the dependent measures of emotional distress. Dependent measures included the Profile of Mood States, an index of vulnerability, the Inventory of Current Concerns (six problem areas), and actual number of physical symptom complaints. Three-fourths of their 133 patients were correctly placed into high or low distress groups, on the basis of pre-treatment MMPI scores.

In conclusion, psychosocial disruption and difficulty in the treatment and re-entry periods has been extensively documented. Not only has a relatively high prevalence of negative affe ts, low self-esteem, and psychosocial dysfunction been established, some investigators have successfully identified poorer post-treatment copers on the basis of pre-treatment symptomatology and personality profile. There is little doubt that the 6-month period after treatment is difficult for a great many patients. The focus of study in this group of patients tends to be on the identification of high risk patients and determination of correlates to psychosocial dysfunction.

Extended survival: psychosocial studies

Many investigators have reported quite favorable overall psychological adjustment to successful cancer treatment [64–66, 85]. Such reports would probably be even more prevalent were it not for the fact that most investigators go into survival studies looking for problems rather than looking for the absence of problems or even positive growth. The result is that these investigations fail to reject the hypothesis that there are no differences between cancer survivors and their age-peers. This is very different from proving that there is no difference. That is, although many studies have failed to detect significant differences between survivors and comparison groups, the nature of hypothesis testing makes it impossible to conclude that differences do not exist. Therefore, investigators continue to search for maladjustment because almost all past studies were designed to either find or 'fail to find' maladjustment.

Examining the prevalence of general post-treatment difficulties, Iszak, Engel, and Medalie [67] surveyed 345 patients, 91 of whom were considered 'cured' at the time of assessment. They found, predictably, that the cured subgroup had the greatest need for vocational services and the lowest need for medical services. Problems identified in the cured group, as assessed by the authors' 'Ability Index' questionnaire, were continued difficulty with physical stamina and with the 'psychological trauma' posed by diagnosis and treatment. Need for social services, including both practical assistance and psychotherapeutic intervention, was acknowledged in 33% of 345 patients [67].

A similar study of psychosocial problems acknowledged by 810 patients off-treatment for an average of 2.5 years found 93% of them still struggling with problems of fatigue [68]. Of this 93%, one in five viewed the fatigue to be incapacitating. The authors speculate that the absence of any identifiable physiological reason for this high figure may provide indirect evidence for lethargy as a depressive equivalent. All patients were over 45, 70% were women, and around half had either breast or uterine cancer. Patient historical accounts revealed an apparent 6-month lag from treatment cessation to the development of depressive symptoms, again suggesting gradual relaxation of defenses [cf. 45, 47]. Sexual dysfunction was the most frequently cited marital problem (47 of 567 married subjects). Other problems included spouse anger or fear of cancer, financial difficulty, spouse withdrawal or spouse alcoholism. While 23% complained of deterioration in their family role satisfaction, 35% claimed their situation had improved as a result of their cancer experience. Health and life insurance readjustments were problematic for 24% of the patients. The percentage of patients employed dropped significantly, from 54 to 47%.

The areas of work discrimination and work adjustment have received a good deal of attention. The available evidence on work discrimination is split between reports of little or no overt or covert discrimination toward the cured cancer patient [69, 70], and assertions of both outright [71] and subtle [72] work and hiring discrimination. In an American Cancer Society study, out of 130 of the most employable recovered cancer patients (age 25–50, employed at the time of diagnosis, and skilled), 22% reported one or more job rejections. Many on-the-job reports of subtle mistreatment such as hostility from co-workers, unnecessary transfers to encourage resignation, lack of salary advances and health benefit rejection were common [72].

Research on work adjustment in post-treatment patients also has shown mixed results. For example, Gordon et al. found one-third of 136 patients off treatment to be experiencing vocational adjustment difficulties [73], while Wheatley et al. found 74 off-treatment cancer patients to be no different from other employees at the Metropolitan Life Insurance Company in absenteism, turnover, job performance, or insurance costs [74]. Not one of the patients was fired for any reason. They had been off treatment for a range of 1 month to 25 years. One explanation for this difference between study findings could be the method of data collection: Gordon et al. used patient self-report while the Wheatley study used employer records. Perhaps the patient experiences a sense of difficulty in adjusting which is not easily detected by gross measures of work performance kept by employers. Alternately, it could be that the patients truly are adjusting well, and their subjective sense of maladjustment might represent a more non-specific problem of general distress. Further study is needed to address this issue.

Schonfield [63] has attempted to predict those patients who will experience post-treatment work readjustment difficulty. In his study of 42 male and female patients, using 63 items of the MMPI and an anxiety questionnaire given before starting treatment, he demonstrated that pre-treatment anxiety (especially about situational concerns) and a low morale loss score on the MMPI were good predictors of later difficulty returning to work. All but nine of 42 patients returned to work within 9 months of treatment. Stage of disease and severity of treatment were not effective predictors of successful return to work.

In a more general study, Mages and Mendelsohn [75] examined 60 patients with various cancer sites, most of whom had received only radiation. Some of these patients were 3- to 6-year survivors. Their findings indicated marked increases in self-image, values and physical capacities over time, but little change in level of dysphoria on the Gough-Heilbrun Adjective Checklist. They also reported improvements in distractibility, absentmindedness and concentration, as well as an increase in focus on home and family concerns over time..Women were more able than men to preserve their sense of self-esteem over time off treatment. The authors comment that in their young adult patients, the cancer experience impeded the development of their self-sufficiency and resulted in delay and disruption of the smooth establishing of adult roles.

Kennedy, Tellegen, Kennedy, and Havernick [76] examined 22 cancer patients (various sites), aged 20–69, 5–20 years off treatment. They found the men to have a significantly higher mean stress-reactivity level on the Differential Personality Questionnaire. Women had a higher mean social closeness score. That is, women particularly valued close and friendly personal relationships, while the men appeared at higher risk for post-treatment distress. Interestingly, all their cancer patients showed a greater appreciation for life, people, time, and interpersonal relationships when compared to matched samples of chronic diabetes patients and normal (healthy) controls. They were less concerned with the 'non-essentials' of life. The authors conclude that cancer, when met with successful treatment, is a good catalyst for character development. They base this conclusion on the finding of generally positive adjustment without significant psychosocial distress, as measured by physician assessment, semantic differential ratings, the Differential Personality Questionnaire, and unstructured interview [76].

Based upon data from unstructured interviews of 20 patients 1–33 years post-diagnosis, Shanfield [77] concluded that fear of cancer, then fear of significant interpersonal loss, were the numbers one and two concerns, respectively, of the surviving cancer patient. Mild depression was detected in 25% of the sample. Physical vulnerability was named as a consequence related to the fear of recurrence. Shanfield also identified a sense of existential resolution with death and life appreciation which the successfully treated patient feels.

Extended survival: psychosexual studies

Psychosexual dysfunction has been reported in cancer survivors as a result of illness residua [79–81], treatment late-effects [82, 83], and interpersonal disruption [84–88]. Prevalence figures of dissatisfaction or dysfunction in sexual areas have ranged from 20–90% [89]. In concluding her excellent review of this area, Andersen [89] asks the following question, each phrase of which pinpoints a critical variable needing further investigation: 'What disease/treatment contexts produce what kind of sexual difficulties for which subgroups of cancer patients over what time course, and what are the etiologic components?' (p. 1839).

In accord with other studies [68, 77] Sutherland [78] identified the fear of rejection as the main source of anxiety in the off-treatment cancer patient. This fear of rejection or abandonment can show itself through sexual dysfunction. Golden and Golden [88] have suggested that the frequently observed desexualization of the cancer patient is often an interpersonal (rather than personal) dysfunction in that it is often the healthy partner who initiates, or at least actively colludes with, disengagement.

Many authors [e.g., 90] have emphasized the primary influence of psychological rather than physiological causes for impotence and general sexual dysfunction in cancer patients. There is some support for this assertion in that sexual dysfunctions often continue well into the post-treatment period, virtually nullifying the possibility of drug- or disease-related etiology. These reported post-treatment dysfunctions have been attributed to decreased libido, concern over performance, defective body image, fear of rejection, gender identity disturbance, fear of disease contagion, and depression [13, 87, 90–92].

In summary of previous investigations of cancer survival, many of the studies on mixed diagnostic groups have been quite extensive with regard to sample size, but very global in the type of inquiry. Previous studies have tended to focus on the presence of general depressive symptomatology and quality of life as reflected in self-report measures. Findings have been inconsistent, due in part to differing methodologies and unclear criteria for 'disturbance'. Research reports on the impact of cancer in the survival period have run the full gamut of conclusions, from positive character growth through no significant change to heightened risk of depression, anxiety, fatigue, work maladjustment and discrimination, and interpersonal difficulties. The growing body of research seems to favor a conservative conclusion, that cancer survival is not associated with major psychosocial disruption, and that it often provides an opportunity to enhance life appreciation. Claims of post-treatment psychosexual dysfunction in the general cancer population have been more impressionistic and superficially documented than carefully empirical. Systematic exploration of this particular area is generally lacking but improving. Some promise is evident in studies of survivors of breast cancer, Hodgkin's disease, and some childhood malignancies such as ALL. These specific areas will now be reviewed briefly.

Breast cancer patients

The fact that breast cancer, if detected early, has long been amenable to successful treatment has led to extensive psychological study of survival in patients with this disease. The insult of cancer upon such a culturally valued sexual body part can have potentially far-reaching psychosexual ramifications. The following studies are representative of the many studies of psychological adjustment to breast cancer survival. Characteristic of research in this area, these studies reveal a pattern of mixed results.

Over the past 20 years, for both medical and cultural reasons, there has been a dramatic shift away from radical mastectomy to modified mastectomy and, more recently, to lumpectomy plus radiation ('breast-sparing' treatment). Because of current uncertainty as to relative long-term efficacy of modified mastectomy versus lumpectomy plus radiation, many women are either choosing one or the other, or agreeing to clinical oncology trials in which they are randomized to one or the other form of treatment. This situation presents us with the opportunity to examine psychological and psychosexual adjustment differences between women who have these very different forms of treatment.

Although the data are mixed, there is an emerging picture of differences between women who have lumpectomy plus radiation and those who have mastectomy. They tend not to differ in areas of psychological symptoms or mood states during the survival period. Gross measures of marital or social satisfaction also tend to be unaffected. However, in areas of body image and sexuality, the woman with lumpectomy seem to feel consistently better [59, 105–107]. Contrary to what might be an intuitive position, the data seem at this point to favor the conclusion that breast-conserving lumpectomy is not associated with heightened fear of recurrence [106, 107]; in fact, this fear may even be higher in mastectomy patients [108].

There are a number of large-scale studies of breast survival which did not address the question of differential adjustment according to treatment, but looked at prevalence of general problems. For example Eisenberg and Goldenberg [42] tested 252 breast cancer patients immediately after mastectomy and 18 months later. They found persistent decrements in self-esteem and an actual drop over time in the percentage of patients who held a positive attitude toward their future, from 54 down to 39%. This drop may represent a lifting of defenses in the recovery phase of survival.

In a mail survey of 826 breast cancer patients randomly selected from the Memorial Hospital registry of 5,472 patients treated for breast cancer between 1949–1962, 84% of survivors off treatment for 5 or more years had, by their own criteria, fully resumed their premorbid lifestyles [93]. Many of this group (14%) said that it took them over 6 months to do so. This suggests that around 30% of these patients failed to successfully resume premorbid functioning within 6 months of completing treatment. Comparing 5-year survivors to 10- and 15-year survivors, they found that severity of disease slowed down the process of return to earlier occupational status: within the 5-year group only, ratings of women with regionally spread disease were lower than those with localized disease.

A very well-controlled study has compared 134 breast cancer patients, most of whom were 5 or more years off treatment, to 139 age-matched controls and 121 neighborhood controls [94]. All were given the same 28-item general health and quality of life questionnaire. There were no significant differences in level of employment, attitude toward life, view of the future, leisure activities, or psychiatric symptoms. The only differences between groups were that the cancer patients rated their current health as poorer and rated themselves as more physically disabled than the two control groups. As these differences have clearly realistic bases, they were not seen as signs of maladjustment in these women.

A prospective investigation, using the 'Ability Index' from an earlier study [95], followed 221 breast cancer patients over a 3-year off-treatment period [83]. All patients, including 90 with stage I and 131 with stage II disease, had the same treatment: radical mastectomy plus radiation. One year after treatment, 201 (91%) were still living; 167 (75%) were still alive at 3 years. General problems surveyed by the Ability Index included subjective complaints about medical treatment, reduced ability to support themselves, change in relationships with family and friends, and emotional well-being vis-à-vis health concerns. Comparing the results at 1 year with those at 3 years off treatment, they identified a slight drop (21 to 15%) in patients with ambulatory limitations, increases in sexual disturbances over time (12 to 18% frequency), improvement in ability to support oneself financially over time (30% disabled to 20% disabled), and a slight drop in social extrafamilial) contact over time. There was no change noted in family relationships over time, lending support to the common notion that one aspect of adaptation to cancer survival entails some withdrawal from the milieu of friends and increased focus on family togetherness. About one in four patients at both times of assessment demonstrated difficulties in lack of self-confidence, fear, frustration, and anger about the future.

In the above study, there was some indication of life enhancement from the cancer experience, but somewhat more evidence for mild psychosocial disruption. Another study has supported this figure of 25% psychological distress after 1 year off treatment, but asserts that this figure drops over the following 4 years [96]. Morris, Greer, and White [62], on the other hand, reported that 30% of their 69 breast patients were psychologically distressed 1 year after treatment. This figure did not drop in the second year. They used psychological tests and a different structured interview, so the different measures and different criteria for distress (interview report vs. test scores) could explain why one group found this drop and the other did not. The study by Morris et al. compared 69 breast cancer patients to 91 women with benign breast disease both cross-sectionally and longitudinally. Two years after diagnosis and surgery, 83% of the cancer group and 76% of the benign group had successfully resumed premorbid work and marital functioning.

A final study examined 49 post-mastectomy patients 4 years after treatment [84]. Through structured interview it was determined that women who complained of more physical symptoms during and after treatment also were in greater psychological distress. Prevalence of sexual dysfunction remained high 4 years off treatment for these women, and was related to marital discord. The authors conclude that social support (including family and social service assistance) has a buffering effect upon the psychosocial adjustment difficulties of the cured breast cancer patient.

Hodgkin's disease patients

In the study of Hodgkin's disease patients off treatment, the emphasis has been on psychosexual adaptation, since the known sterilizing effects of combination chemotherapy and radiation have led oncologists to be concerned about psychosexual dysfunction which might arise. Again, the research in this area has yielded mixed findings.

In conjunction with their initial trials of MOPP chemotherapy, Sherins and DeVita [97] found that 16 treated Hodgkin's disease patients experienced normal ejaculation despite abnormal spermatogenesis. In a larger study, 74 Hodgkin's disease patients were assessed an average of 27 months after treatment [82]. Compared to a rate of 74% during treatment, 46% of all patients complained of decreased libido and sexual performance in the post-treatment period. Few of this 46% were subjectively distressed about their difficulty, however. Six of 54 men were rendered impotent. Four of these cases had no physiological basis for their impotence.

In a related study [98], 47 male Hodgkin's patients were asked about general quality of life and subjective personality changes as well as psychosexual dysfunction. Most of these patients were studied prospectively, from the pre-treatment period through treatment cessation. Twenty-one of them were post-treatment patients who made retrospective ratings of the treatment and survival periods. Half of all patients stated their libido had not returned to pre-treatment levels. They did, however, acknowledge a gradual increase in libido and general quality of life over the years while in complete remission. Other findings of the study included a tendency toward increase in violent behavior and irritability in the post-treatment period. Irritability, for example, was given as a 'status quo' affect in 84% of patients recently off treatment, as opposed to 16% of pre-treatment patients. The authors concluded that the emotional response of a young man becoming ill may represent a particular vulnerability in that the dependency of illness and the sterilizing effect of treatment are decidedly 'unmasculine' experiences which can challenge the smooth transition into adulthood.

In a larger study [99], 156 male Hodgkin's patients, ranging from 43–141 months off treatment, were interviewed. Most of them were between the ages of 15–40. Using gross career criteria and patient comparisons of lifestyle changes contrasting retrospective pre-treatment ratings to current ratings, the authors concluded that nearly all of the sample had led 'normal' post-treatment lives. Of 263 (male *and* female) patients, four had severe physical complications and only two displayed serious psychiatric disturbance.

The 'MOPP' (Nitrogen Mustard, Oncovin, Procarbazine, Prednisone) chemotherapy regimen used with Hodgkin's disease has tremendous emetogenic potential. The presence of anticipatory nausea and vomiting in patients during the course of treatment has been known for some time. However, it is now becoming apparent that the aversive conditioning in many patients receiving MOPP and other emetogenic drugs (e.g., cisplatinum), persists for years after treatment. In a study of 60 Hodgkin's disease survivors 6–120 months post chemotherapy, over half complained of persistent anticipatory nausea [104]. The cues associated with this nausea were usually smells reminiscent of the treatment ordeal (e.g., rubbing alcohol, hospital cleaning solutions, perfumes worn by staff, etc.), or sights such as the hospital or treatment room, encountered at follow-up visits. Follow-up appointments in general have been reported as problematic for surviving patients [85, 104]. What remains unknown is whether the fear and general distress aroused by the prospect of follow-up visits cause problems with compliance or self-monitoring in the off-treatment period.

In a study comparing 37 Hodgkin's disease patients aged 18–45 to young adult parents of leukemic children [100], the parent group was shown to have greater overall psychological distress. Of the 37 Hodgkin's patients, 32 were off treatment for 2 or more years ($M = 5.5$ years). Both the parents and the 32 Hodgkin's patients more than 2 years off treatment had higher anxiety scores on the Gottschalk-Gleser [101] Content Analysis Scale than the scale's normative sample. Unlike the parent group, however, the Hodgkin's patients did not score any higher than the normative sample on level of hostility.

Survivors of childhood malignancies: 'The Damocles Syndrome'

The realization that no study had comprehensively assessed mental health or psychological adjustment in childhood cancer survivors led Koocher et al. to initiate extensive investigation of this area [15, 57, 102]. Koocher and O'Malley's book, titled 'The Damocles Syndrome' [15], takes its name from the story of Damocles, who was forced to sit at a banquet in the court of Dionysus under a sword suspended by a single hair, to depict the precariousness of his fortunes. Such uncertainty is presented by the authors as the dilemma which all successfully treated cancer patients face during the initial years following treatment, if not for their entire lives. The book presents the results of an intensive examination of 117 childhood cancer survivors and a comparison group of 22 children with various chronic diseases. The children with cancer included patients with neuroblastoma, leukemia, osteosarcoma, non-Hodgkin's lymphoma, or Hodgkin's disease. Mean age at diagnosis was 5.5 years, and mean age at testing was 18. All children were at least 5 years post-diagnosis.

The authors of the study identified 'uncertainty of survival' as the chief independent variable. Thus, they did not play close attention to time off treatment or disease severity as potential factors. They did, however, compare different diagnostic categories to each other on some of the measures. Dependent measures were administered to all subjects and included a combined adjustment rating scale, a standardized interview including mental status examination, a standardized psychiatric interview for children, the Wechsler Intelligence Scale's Information, Similarities and Vocabulary subtests, the Vineland Social Maturity Scale, a self-rating depression scale, a death anxiety questionnaire, a short form of the Taylor Manifest Anxiety Scale, a self-esteem measure, and TAT cards 1, 3GF, 8BM, 13B, and 14 as well as four drawings of hospital scenes. These nine stories were scored for content reflecting sadness, loneliness, individual reflection, and story resolution.

The principal finding of their study was that 47% of 117 long-term survivors of childhood cancer showed some degree of adjustment difficulty as measured by the combined adjustment ratings of two independent raters. This percentage was significantly greater than that for the smaller group of children with chronic illness. Within the cancer group, the highest prevalence of adjustment difficulty was in the Hodgkin's disease subgroup (64%). The authors proposed two interpretations for this. One was that because this was the oldest subgroup of patients, it may indicate that psychosocial adjustment to childhood cancer is more problematic for older children and adolescents than for younger children. This makes intuitive sense in that the developmental tasks of adolescence are in direct opposition to the dependency which sickness and recovery engender. The second interpretation offered was that the more prolonged treatment which Hodgkin's disease patients receive by comparison to other childhood cancers may increase the sense of uncertainty and danger which the young patient experiences. Many Hodgkin's patients undergo splenectomies which can prolong immunodeficiencies. Successfully treated Hodgkin's patients may therefore be required to take antibiotics prophylactically long after treatment ends; an ever present reminder of continued vulnerability. This question of age versus treatment effects upon cancer survival is an important one which demands more empirical attention.

In this same investigation no differences were found between the general cancer group and the chronic illness comparison group in verbal intelligence or social maturity [15]. Likewise, cancer patients did not show elevated death anxiety, manifest anxiety, or depression. Self-esteem as measured by self-report was not significantly lower. Multiple regression analysis showed higher intelligence and higher socio-economic status were good predictors of positive adjustment. As implied earlier, age at diagnosis was also a good predictor of positive adjustment, with younger patients faring better. Time since diagnosis, while not built into the hypotheses of the study, did show itself to be a good predictor of adjustment (the more time elapsed, the better). Disease severity did not.

Koocher and O'Malley conclude their book with a formulation of adaptation to cancer based upon their empirical findings and their review of the literature. They conclude that the 'stress' of cancer is greatest at the point of diagnosis and initiation of treatment, and that it slowly diminishes over time, nearly reaching baseline at 5 years post-diagnosis. During the course of this decline, various events such as recurrence, symptom distress or death in the family can disturb the settling process and initiate elevations in stress. The patient, in a state of heightened vulnerability due to the protracted working through of the impact of cancer and its treatment, is likely to be more easily over-excited and distressed. This, according to the authors, is optimally dealt with through adaptive denial which is best described as a conscious suppression of feelings, and an increase in activity to counterbalance the passivity of illness. The almost universal use of some denial, in 99 % of patients [102] is again a powerful testimony to its effectiveness if not necessity.

Conclusion

In general, the research on cancer survival has yielded mixed results. Quite often, protracted and exaggerated psychological symptomatology such as depression, anxiety, somatization, fatigue, and irritability have been reported. Evidence for significant psychosexual dysfunction, particularly as it is affected by body image and interpersonal concerns, has been presented. Psychosocial areas of occupational functioning and marital satisfaction have also been cited as problematic. On the other hand, there are investigators who deny the presence of significant psychosocial or psychosexual disruption in the cancer survivor. Some have even emphasized the positive, growthful aspects of having suffered through and endured the ordeal of successful cancer treatment. In some studies, both positive and negative effects have been reported to coexist, possibly exerting separate influences upon adaptation.

There are several problems with most previous investigations which may contribute to the inconsistencies and inconclusiveness of the results outlined. First, investigations have differed greatly in their use of control or comparison groups. Some have used no comparison group at all, opting to compare their findings to established base rates, normative data, or mere common sense. Second, measurement of dependent variables has often been global, and has tended to rely upon non-standardized interview responses rather than structured questionnaires or more in-depth projective tests. A third problem is that the cancer groups being studied in the past have often been quite heterogeneous. Of those studies which have examined isolated disease sites, the separate effects of age, treatment severity, or length of time off treatment have usually been minimal or non-existent. Therefore, more extensive study of cancer survival, focusing on specific diagnostic groups, specific treatment regimens, and clearly delineated survival periods is necessary to help clarify the specific psychosocial problems and sequelae in cancer survival.

Certainly the psychological cost of successful cancer treatment is greatly outweighed by the benefit of extended life. The goals of research in this area are to identify the extent to which quality of life in survival is associated with differing sites and treatments; to identify patients who can be expected to show distress during survival; and to help inform comprehensive treatment planners about what issues to anticipate in the growing number of surviving cancer patients.

References

1. Holland JC. 1981. The humanistic side of cancer care: Changing issues and challenges. Proceedings of the American Cancer Society, Third National Conference on Human Values and Cancer, pp 1–13.
2. American Cancer Society. 1985. Cancer facts and figures. American Cancer Society, New York.
3. National Cancer Institute. 1984. Surveillance, Epidemiology, and End Results Program (SEER). Annual Cancer Statistics Review, November.
4. Blumberg R, Flaherty M, Lewis J. (eds). 1980. Coping with cancer. U.S. Department of Health and Human Services, National Institutes of Health, NIH Publication No. 80–2080, September.
5. D'Angio GJ, Ross JW. 1981. The cured cancer patient: A new problem in attitudes and communication. Proceedings of the American Cancer Society Third National Conference on Human Values and Cancer, pp 34–49.
6. Katz J, Weiner H, Gallagher T, Hellman L. 1970. Stress, distress and ego defenses, psychoendocrine response to impending breast tumor biopsy. Arch Gen Psych 23:131–142.
7. Lipowski A. 1970. Physical illness, the individual and the coping processes. Int J Psych Med 1(2):91–102.
8. Cohen F, Lazarus R. 1973. Active coping processes, coping dispositions, and recovery from surgery. Psychosom Med 35:375–389.
9. Janis I. 1958. Psychological stress. Wiley, New York.
10. Silberfarb PM. 1982. Research in adaptation to illness and psychosocial intervention: An overview. Proceedings of the Working Conference on the Psychological, Social, and Behavioral Medicine Aspects of Cancer: Research and Professional Education Needs and Directions for the 1980's. American Cancer Society, pp 1921–1925.
11. Silberfarb P, Maurer L, Crouthamel C. 1980. Psychosocial aspects of neoplastic disease: I. Functional status of breast cancer patients during different treatment regimens. Am J Psych 137(4):450–455.
12. Holland J, Rowland J, Lebovits A, Rusalem R. 1979. Reactions to cancer treatment: Assessment of emotional response to adjuvant radiotherapy as a guide to planned intervention. Psych Clin North Am 2(29):347–358.
13. Sutcliffe SB. 1979. Cytoxic chemotherapy and gonadal function in patients with Hodgkin's disease: Facts and thoughts. J Am Med Assoc 242(17):1898–1899.
14. Kagen-Goodheart L. 1977. Re-entry: Living with childhood cancer. Am J Orthopsych 47:651–658.
15. Koocher G, O'Malley J. 1981. The Damocles Syndrome: Psychosocial consequences of surviving childhood cancer. McGraw-Hill, New York.
16. Penman D. 1979. Coping strategies in adaptation to mastectomy. Yeshiva University: Unpublished doctoral dissertation.
17. Worden W, Sobel H. 1978. Ego strength and psychosocial adaptation to cancer. Psychosom Med 40(8):585–592.

168

18. Sobel H, Worden W. 1979. The MMPI as a predictor of psychosocial adaptation to cancer. J Consult Clin Psychol 37(4):716-724.
19. Freidenbergs I, Gordon W, Hibbard M, Levine L, Wolf C, Diller L. 1981-82. Psychosocial aspects of living with cancer: A review of the literature. Int J Psych Med 11(4):303-329.
20. Holland J. 1982. Psychologic aspects of cancer. In: Cancer medicine. Holland JF, Frei E (eds). Lea & Febiger, Philadelphia.
21. Weisman A. 1976. Early diagnosis of vulnerability in cancer patients. Am J Med Sci 271:187.
22. Sutherland, A, Orbach CE, Dyk RB. 1952. Psychological impact of cancer and cancer surgery. I. Adaptation to dry colostomy: Preliminary report and summary of findings. Cancer 5:857-872.
23. Sutherland A. 1956. Psychological impact of cancer and its therapy. Med Clin North Am 40:705-720.
24. Bard M, Sutherland AM. 1955. Psychological impact of cancer and its treatment. IV. Adaptation to radical mastectomy. Cancer 8:656-672.
25. Caplan G. Mastery of stress: Psychosocial aspects. Am J Psych 138(4):413-420.
26. Horowitz M. 1976. Stress response syndromes. Aronson, New York.
27. Lindemann E. 1944. Symptomatology and management of acute grief. J Psych 101:141-148.
28. Horowitz MJ. 1982. Stress response syndromes and their treatment. In: Handbook of stress: Theoretical and clinical aspects. Goldberger L, Breznitz S (eds). Macmillan, New York.
29. Taylor SE. 1983. Adjustment to threatening events: A theory of cognitive adaptation. Am Psychol 38:1161-1173.
30. Taylor SE. 1984 Attributions, beliefs about control, and adjustment to breast cancer. J Personal Soc Psychol 46:489-502.
31. Nerenz DR, Coons HL, Lasky G, Leventhal H, Love RR. 1984. Adjustment to threatening events: Cancer chemotherapy. Paper presented at the 92nd annual Convention of the American Psychological Association, Toronto.
32. Lehrman DR, Wortman CB, Williams AF. Long-term effects of losing a spouse or child in a motor vehicle crash. J Personal Soc Psychol (in press).
33. Wortman CB. 1983. Coping with victimization: Conclusions and implications for future research. J Soc Iss 39, 2:197-223.
34. Taplin J. 1971. Crisis theory: Critique and reformulation. Comm Ment Health J 7:13-23.
35. Lewis M, Gottesman D, Gutstein S. 1979. The course and duration of crisis. J Consult Clin Psychol 47:128-134.
36. Gottesman D, Lewis M. 1982. Differences in crisis reactions among cancer and surgery patients. J Consult Clin Psychol 50(3):381-388.
37. Sveinson K. 1977. Learning to live with cancer. Martin's Press, New York.
38. Zubrod C. 1975. Successes in cancer treatment. Cancer 36:267-270.
39. Bronner-Huszar J. 1971. The psychological aspects of cancer in man. Psychosomatics 12:133-138.
40. Cohen M, Wellisch D. 1978. Living in limbo: Psychosocial intervention in families with a cancer patient. Am J Psych 32:561-571.
41. McCollum P. 1978. Adjustment to cancer: A psychosocial and rehabilitation perspective. Rehabil Couns Bull 21:216-223.
42. Eisenberg H, Goldenberg I. 1966. A measurement of quality of survival of breast cancer patients. In: Clinical evaluation in breast cancer: Symposium on clinical evaluation in breast cancer, London, 1965. Hayward J. Bulbrook R (eds). Academic Press, New York.

43. Gorzynski G, Holland J. 1979. Psychological aspects of testicular cancer. Sem Oncol 6:25–29.
44. Clapp MJ. 1976. Psychosocial reactions of children with cancer. Nurs Clin North Am 11:73–82.
45. Spinetta J, Maloney L. 1975. Death anxiety in the outpatient leukemic child. Pediatrics 56:1034–1037.
46. Hackett T, Weisman A. 1969. Denial as a factor in patients with heart disease and cancer. Ann N Y Acad Sci 164:802–811.
47. O'Neill M. 1975. Psychological aspects of cancer recovery. Cancer 36:271–273.
48. Weisman A, Worden JW. 1976–77. The existential plight in cancer: Significance of the first 100 days. Int J Psych Med 7(1):1–15.
49. Gordon W, Freidenbergs I, Diller L, Hibbard, Levine L, Wolf C, Ezrachi O, Lipkins T. 1979. The effects of psychosocial intervention on cancer patients. Paper presented at the 87th American Psychological Association Convention, New York.
50. Chodoff P, Friedman B, Hamburg D. 1964. Stress, defenses and coping behavior: Observations in parents of children with malignant disease. Am J Psych 120:743–749.
51. Levy S. 1984. The process and outcome of 'adjustment' in the cancer patient: A reply to Taylor. Am Psychol 39:1327.
52. Derogatis L, Abeloff M, Melisaratos N. 1979. Psychological coping mechanisms and survival time in metastatic breast cancer. J Am Med Assoc 241:1504–1508.
53. Rogentine G, Van Kammen D, Fox B, Rosenblatt J, Docherty J, Barney W. 1978. Psychological and biological factors in the prognosis of melanoma. Paper presented at the 86th American Psychological Association Convention, Toronto.
54. Pettingale KW, Morris T, Greer S, Haybittle JL. 1985. Mental attitudes to cancer: An additional prognostic factor. Lancet March 30:750.
55. Fox BH. 1983. Current theory of psychogenic effects on cancer incidence and prognosis. J Psychosoc Oncol 1:17–21.
56. Cassileth BR, Lusk EJ, Miller DS, Brown LL, Miller C. 1985. Psychosocial correlates of survival in advanced malignant disease? New Engl J Med 312(24):1551–1555.
57. Koocher G, O'Malley J, Gogan J, Foster D. 1980. Psychological adjustment among pediatric cancer survivors. J Child Psychol Psych 21:163–173.
58. Weisman A. 1975. Psychosocial analysis of cancer deaths. Omega 6:61–75.
59. Marshall JR, Funch DP. 1983. Social environment and breast cancer: A cohort analysis of patient survival. Cancer 52:1546–1550.
60. Weisman A, Worden JW. 1977. Coping and vulnerability in cancer patients. Research report funded by the National Cancer Institute.
61. Myerowitz B, Sparks F, Spears I. 1979. Adjuvant chemotherapy for breast carcinoma; Psychosocial implications. Cancer 43:1613–1618.
62. Morris T, Greer H, White P. 1977. Psychological and social adjustment to mastectomy. Cancer 40:2381–2387.
63. Schonfield J. 1972. Psychological factors related to delayed return to an earlier life-style in successfully treated cancer patients. J Psychosom Res 16:41–46.
64. Brown R, Haddox V, Posada A, Rubio A. 1972. Social and psychological adjustment following pelvic exenteration. Am J Obstet Gynecol 114:162–171.
65. DaRugna D, Buchheim F. 1979. Quality of life, invalidity, and complications after the treatment of gynecologic cancers. Therapeut Umschau 36(6):559–567.
66. Holmes H, Holmes F. 1975. After ten years, what are the handicaps and lifestyles of children treated for cancer? Clin Pediat 14:819–823.
67. Iszak F, Engel J, Medalie J. 1973. Comprehansive rehabilitation of the patient with cancer: Five-year experience of a home-care unit. J Chron Dis 26:363–374.

68. Greenleigh Associates, Inc. 1979 Report on the social, economic, and psychological needs of cancer patients in California: Major findings and implications. American Cancer Society, California Division, San Francisco.

69. Reynolds J. 1977. The employability of work-able cancer patients. Executive summary, findings, conclusions and recommendations: Survey of employers and patients in New York, St. Louis and Houston, University Research Corporation, Washington, D.C.

70. Stone R. 1975. Employing the recovered cancer patient. Cancer 36:285–286.

71. Feldman F. 1978. Work and cancer helath histories. American Cancer Society.

72. American Cancer Society, California Division. Is there equal opportunity for cancer patients? Am Cancer Soc Volunteer 22(2):2–7.

73. Gordon W, Freidenbergs I, Diller L, Hibbard M, Levine, L, Wolf C, Ezrachi O, Francis A. 1977. The psychological problems of cancer patients: A retrospective study. Paper presented at the 85th American Psychological Association Convention, San Francisco.

74. Wheatley G, Cunnick W, Wright B, Van Keuren D. 1974. The employment of persons with a history of treatment of cancer. Cancer 33:441–445.

75. Mages N, Mendelsohn G. 1979. Effects of cancer on patients' lives: A personological approach. In: Health psychology. Stone G, Cohen F, Adler N (eds). Jossey-Bass, San Francisco.

76. Kennedy B, Tellegen A, Kennedy S, Havernick N. 1976. Psychological response of patients cured of advanced cancer. Cancer 38:2184–2191.

77. Shanfield S. 1980. On surviving cancer: Psychological considerations. Comprehens Psych 21(2):128–134.

78. Sutherland A. 1960. The Psychological impact of cancer. American Cancer Society, New York.

79. Kirkpatrick JR. 1979. The stoma patient and his return to society. Front Rad Ther Oncol 14:20–25.

80. Devlin HB, Plant JA, Griffin M. 1971. Aftermath of surgery for anorectal cancer. Br. Med J 3:413–418.

81. de Bernardinis G, Tuscano D, Negro P et al. 1981. Sexual dysfunction in males following extensive anorectal surgery. Int Surg 66:133–135.

82. Chapman R, Sutcliffe S, Rees L, Edwards C, Malpas J. 1979. Cyclical combination chemotherapy and gonadal function: A retrospective study in males. Lancet, February:285–289.

83. Iszak F, Feller B, Brenner H, Medalie J, Tugendreich J. 1975. Assessment of the quality of life of the breast cancer patient. J Israeli Med Assoc 89(10):445–448.

84. Woods NF, Earp I. 1978. Women with cured breast cancer: A study of mastectomy patients in North Carolina. Nurs Res 27(5):279–285.

85. Cella DF, Tross S. Psychological adjustment to survival from Hodgkin's disease. J Consult Clin Psychol (in press).

86. Derogatis L. 1979. Breast and gynecologic cancers: Their unique impact on body image and sexual identity in females. Front Rad Ther Oncol 14:1–11.

87. Schain W. 1982. Sexual problems of patients with cancer. In: Cancer: Principles and practice of oncology. DeVita V, Hellman S. Rosenberg S (eds). Lippincott, Philadelphia.

88. Golden J, Golden M. 1979. Cancer and sex. Front Rad Ther Oncol 14:59–65.

89. Andersen BL. 1985. Sexual functioning morbidity among cancer survivors: Current status and future research directions. Cancer 55:1835–1842.

90. Grinker R. 1976. Sex and cancer. Med Aspects Hum Sex 10:2.

91. Chapman RM. 1982. Effect of cytotoxic therapy on sexuality and gonadal function. Sem Oncol 9(1):84–94.

92. Wise T. 1978. Effects of cancer on sexual activity. Psychosomatics 19(12):769–775.

93. Schottenfeld D, Robbins G. 1970. Quality of survival among patients who have had radical mastectomy. Cancer 26:650–654.

94. Craig T, Comstock G, Geiser P. 1974. The quality of survival in breast cancer: A case-controlled comparison. Cancer 33:1451–1457.
95. Iszak F, Medalie J. 1971. Comprehensive follow-up of carcinoma patinets. J Chron Dis 24:179–191.
96. Maguire G. 1976. The psychological and social sequelae of mastectomy. In: Modern perspectives in the psychological aspects of surgery. Howell G (ed). Brunner-Mazel, New York.
97. Sherins RJ, DeVita VT. 1973. Effect of drug treatment for lymphoma on male reproductive capacity: Studies of men in remission after therapy. Ann Intern Med 79:216–220.
98. Chapman R, Sutcliffe S, Malpas J. 1981. Male gonadal dysfunction in Hodgkin's disease. J Am Med Assoc 245(13):1323–1328.
99. Cunningham J, Mauch P, Rosenthal D, Canellos G. 1982. Long-term complications of MOPP chemotherapy in patients with Hodgkin's disease. Cancer Treat Rep 66(4):1015–1022.
100. Morrow G. 1980. Parental interrelationships in living with pediatric cancer. Proceedings of the First National Conference for Parents of Children with Cancer, NIH Pub. #80-2176, 175–195.
101. Gottschalk L, Gleser G. 1969. The measurement of psychological states through the content analysis of verbal behavior. University of California Press, Berkeley and Los Angeles.
102. O'Malley J, Koocher G, Foster D, Slavin L. 1979. Psychiatric sequelae of surviving childhood cancer. Am J Orthopsych 49(4):608–616.
103. Levy SM, Herberman RB, Maluish AM, Schlein B, Lippman M. 1985. Prognostic risk assessment in primary breast cancer by behavioral and immunological parameters. Health Psychol 4(2):99–113.
104. Cella DF, Pratt A, Holland JC. 1986. Persistent anticipatory nausea, vomiting and anxiety in cured Hodgkin's disease patients after completion of chemotherapy. Am J Psych 143:641–643.
105. Taylor SE, Lichtman RR, Wood J et al. 1985. Illness-related and treatment-related factors in psychological adjustment to Breast cancer. Cancer 55:2506–2513.
106. Steinberg MD, Juliano MA, Wise L. 1985. Psychological outcome of lumpectomy versus mastectomy in the treatment of breast cancer. Am J Psych 142:34–39.
107. Schain W, Edwards BK, Gorell CR et al. 1983. Psychosocial and physical outcome of primary breast cancer therapy: Mastectomy vs. excisional biopsy and irradiation. Breast Cancer Res Treat 3:377–382.
108. Bartelink H, VanDam F, VanDongen J. 1985. Psychological effects of breast conserving therapy in comparison with radical mastectomy. Rad Oncol Biol Phys 11:381–385.

11. Hospice care

SANDRA JACOBY KLEIN

Abstract

In the past 10–12 years there have been many articles addressing issues in the living/dying process that accompanies the final phase of life. Many of them deal with hospice care – a specialized care for the terminally ill and their significant others. Some controversy surrounding this type of care arises from (1) the difficulty of scientifically evaluating significant qualities such as enthusiasm, devotion, caring and frankness (in discussing death) and (2) the ambiguity and inconsistency of human reactions to dying. Nevertheless the rapid growth of this service suggests that previously ignored needs are now being addressed.

This chapter seeks to offer the reader a brief background on the concept of hospice and the variety of facilities available, the importance of understanding the psychosocial needs of patients and their families, guidelines for physicians caring for the terminally ill and some evaluation research findings.

Background

In the course of the 20th century dying has changed in 'some of the most industrialized, urbanized and technologically advanced areas of the Western World' and death has become 'medicalized' [1]. Starting very discreetly in the 1930s and 40s, becoming widespread after 1950, death in most cases occurred in the hospital. Rapid advances in comfort, privacy, personal hygiene and ideas about asepsis have made everyone more sensitive to sights, smells and sufferings that were once part of daily life. Now these are no longer tolerated.

Once a terminal prognosis is made and the final stage of the illness approaches, the standard procedure is to remove the patient from familiar surroundings and to utilize a hospital or convalescent home for the final

Higby, DJ (ed), Issues in Supportive Care of Cancer Patients. ISBN 0-89838-816-3.
© *1986, Martinus Nijhoff Publishers, Boston. Printed in the Netherlands.*

days of life. The dying person is placed in a distant room where he/she is, for the most part, uninvolved in daily life. The nurses manage basic needs, most treatment stops and the physician tends to make quick, infrequent visits. These settings become the places of the normal death, expected and accepted by all. 'The dying man's bedroom has passed from the home to the hospital' [1].

One noticeable factor in the medicalization of death is the increased life span of the terminally ill due to advances in medical treatment. This makes both the length of the patient's life questionable and difficult to predict, and also heightens the expectance of the loss. The significant other and the patient have to deal with not only the diagnosis but also with the slow-motion movement of the disease. Everyone is held in limbo – physically and psychosocially.

As the disease drags on, often becoming a chronic illness punctuated by acute episodes needing supportive services, the stress and strain increase. Peripheral caregivers drop away tending to leave one significant other to carry the burden. This person frequently undergoes enormous physical and emotional strain often experiencing feelings of helplessness, hostility, resentment and depression. The stress and strain on this individual can be manifested in various ways including sleep disorders, erratic eating habits and changes in the social relationships that once offered support.

Another factor in the medicalization of death is the increase in the time that the patient spends in the hospital. Medical expertise, competent personnel, surgical advances and lengthy medical treatments generally have led the terminally ill to be repeatedly admitted to the hospital. The significant others, believing that the hospital and its staff are more expert than they in caring for the patient's needs, shift the burden of care, gratefully and seemingly without guilt. Many begin to feel convinced that they are inadequate as caregivers. By giving up their roles, they begin to be excluded from the living/dying process. Yet, once acute episodes are resolved and treatments are discontinued, the patient, no longer in need of hospital care, often returns home with or near the significant other. This caregiver, having been excluded from the caregiving during hospitalization, is often ill-prepared to continue any care at home.

As these circumstances occur more and more frequently health professionals have become aware of the need to involve and support the caregivers as well as offering care and support to the patients. On many occasions the needs of the family outweigh the needs of the patient [2]. The family is affected at all levels by terminal illness: individually, as a group and in its relation to society [3]. It has also become quite clear that guidelines for involving people in the care are not available nor are medical schools teaching about death and dying in a way that will aid their students in handling these circumstances.

Even though most clinicians are beginning to recognize the impact of the death on the survivors, clinical studies have continued to be done with the dying patient in the hospital setting during times when the family members are usually excluded. Nonetheless as more and more of these studies are published, the results suggest that there is a point in the life cycle at which technology reaches its limitations and the importance of human relationships must be acknowledged. It has become apparent that keeping a patient alive at all costs is not always appropriate, economically feasible or sensitive to the needs of the patient and/or the family.

The health care delivery system does not seem to be responding effectively to these issues. The time has come to find an alternative way for the dying patient to approach the final stages of illness and impending death. This alternative also has to provide necessary support for the family. The hospice movement attempts to address these needs.

History of the hospice movement

In 1967 in the suburbs of London, a place was established that would become the model for an alternative health care delivery system in the living/dying process. St. Christopher's Hospice was established by Dr. Cicely Saunders, who was concerned with the quality of remaining life in a recognized terminally ill patient. The aim of hospice is to make this remaining time as full and comfortable as possible. Dr. Saunders states that 'terminal illness is a time for reconciliation and fulfillment for patient and family and may well be the most important period they spend together' [4]. Death is recognized as part of life and hospice care strives to facilitate a natural flow from life to death. Hospice also strives to create an environment where fear of dying doesn't spoil joy in living [5].

In 1975 this method arrived in the United States with the opening of the New Haven Hospice in Connecticut. The growth of hospice here has been steady and by October 1985 the National Hospice Organization (NHO) recorded 1367 hospices. This rapid growth might be accounted for by underlying social changes such as: a better definition of and new attitudes toward death, a general dissatisfaction with the health care delivery system, more emphasis on self-care, emphasis on treating the whole patient and the passage of federal hospice legislation in 1982 [6].

Hospice concept and goals

At the present time most hospice programs care for terminally ill cancer patients. However, implicit in the concept is the availability of care to any patient with a terminal or progressive illness when acute care facilities no longer have anything to offer. The unit of care is the family. Individual, cultural and psychosocial needs of this unit are recognized and considered. The main goal of hospice care is to see that the patient lives life to the fullest possible potential while being provided with efficient, loving care.

Emphasis is placed on pain and symptom control as opposed to cure. Patients are spared the discomfort of diagnostic procedures and ancillary studies unless they are needed to control symptoms or relieve pain. There is no concern that the patient will become 'addicted' to pain medications and it is generally well-known by physicians that round-the-clock administration of pain-killing medication can usually be given at a lower dosage than that given only when pain occurs and is intense. Erasing the memory of the pain relieves the patient and family of undue anxiety. When patients suffer less pain, the family is less worried about patient discomfort and tends to be less anxious.

Another major focus of hospice care has been the emotional effect of the illness on the patient and his/her family. Concerns for the psychological as well as the physical trauma of the dying process is a documented feature. This emphasis is articulated in the revised principles and standards of the NHO [7] and has been addressed in assessment of hospice efforts [8].

Another goal of hospice is to facilitate home stays and home deaths for those who desire them. Family members are offered training in attending to the medical and nursing needs of the patient at home. This training is supplemented by regular, frequent calls and visits from the hospice home care team usually consisting of one or more of the following: physician, nurse and/or home health aide, social worker and physical therapist if needed. The offer of relief and support by the home care team helps prevent frequent hospitalizations, thereby eliminating one of the great expenses of long-term illness. The skilled home care team can assess family skills and interactions which contribute to this experience and can advise continued home care or hospitalization. The availability of home care support, as well as hospital care, instills a sense of continuity through the illness.

Demands of home patient care are great and caregivers are assisted in realigning family roles and adapting to an expected loss through the support of the professional staff. Family bonds are often strengthened during this time thus possibly diminishing the severity of post death bereavement [9].

Family members and the patient are all encouraged to be involved in decisions made regarding the patient's treatment. It is thought that this involvement increases their satisfaction with patient care [8, 10]. They are also offered assistance with legal, economic, bureaucratic and spiritual problems associated with terminal illness and death.

If the patient is unable to be cared for in the home then unrestricted visitation and provision of facilities for the family are usually available at the inpatient hospice. The presence of loved ones often helps allay patient fears. A less fearful, relaxed patient tends to prevent increased anxiety in the significant other. This lack of restriction on visiting time also alleviates the patient's sense of isolation and loneliness and eases the family into the realization of the transitions occurring during the final stages. Those who experience the transitions learn to adapt and reconcile the death easier than those who are kept away from the process.

Hospice staffing

The health care delivery approach at most hospices is multidisciplinary. It involves physicians, nurses and mental health professionals in a higher staff/patient ratio than that found in most medical facilities. Trained volunteers are utilized in great numbers in order to decrease costs and offer one-to-one companionship and support to the patient and respite to the family caregivers. Spiritual counseling is also available. This team is most effective when specifically trained to provide care for terminally ill patients and their significant others. Part of their training might include methods of identifying factors of greatest importance to the patient and/or family members. In order to provide optimum care and to satisfy physical, social and emotional needs, it is necessary to understand and identify patient and family needs and interactions [8].

Ideally, the staff draws together in a family-type of group, giving support to each other that is reflected in the approach to the care of the patients and their families. Ongoing support services for health care providers are always made a part of any hospice program. Without this support, burn-out can be quite high in this stressful work.

Commitment by the hospice staff to the patient and family means being involved and not shying away from giving emotional support, counseling, verbal and non-verbal communication and information to alleviate fears. It is most important to coordinate this health care delivery team's services with the services of any other caregivers. This not only enhances the team's skills, but also aids in continuity of care and follow-through of goals. The family, after months of being the main support for the patient finally has a resource for needed assistance and respite.

Hospice models

In the past 10 years hospice concepts and goals have begun to be incorporated into new and existing health care facilities in the United States.

Although inpatient and home care are the two basic settings, there are predominantly five models of service delivery at this time [11]:

1. freestanding, inpatient hospice;
2. hospital-affiliated, freestanding hospice;
3. hospital-based hospice;
   a. centralized palliative care unit,
   b. hospice consultation service circulating in an acute care hospital;
   c. Health Maintenance Organization (HMO) units;
4. hospice within an extended care facility;
5. home health care program;
   a. community based,
   b. hospital based,
   c. nursing home based.

Existing facilities have certain advantages besides their structure. They already have established supportive services such as laundry, laboratory, kitchen, pharmacy and administration; multidisciplinary staffs; and the ability to bill third party payment sources for their services.

The inpatient units often seek to create environments that offer maximum physical and psychological comfort for the patient and family. A complete kitchen is often available for preparation of a patient's favorite foods. Rooms are decorated with items from home such as paintings, photographs, bedspreads and small pieces of furniture. Some facilities provide space for conjugal visits. This environment also supports unrestricted visiting by family members (including children), friends, and favorite pets.

Role of the physician

Cancer symbolizes and is often equated with death in this society [12]. For many types of cancer there is limited therapy which in itself may be toxic. Also, it is difficult for some physicians to consider the discontinuance of active therapy. Physicians are expected to provide care and support that will lead to a cure and dealing with the failure of therapy is disappointing. At the point when this issue arises the only care left to give is palliative care, in which most physicians have had limited training.

This aspect adds an additional challenge to caring for a cancer patient. Cancer care makes special demands on a physician and there are many stories of doctors who withdraw from treating these cases and who become gruff and distant when they can no longer deal with questions asked by patients and family members. Behavioral changes may also occur and might manifest themselves in eating binges; buying sprees; outbursts of anger or sadness; withdrawal; reckless driving and/or substance abuse. Some doctors may become depressed or suicidal when caring for the terminally ill patient.

If the physician can accept him/herself as a human being with human response to these stresses and is willing to seek (psychological) support when needed then he/she will be better able to serve patients.

As part of a multidisciplinary team found in hospice care the physician is going to have less authority and control. For this reason, some have said that hospice programs tend to be anti-doctor or do not need or value active medical participation [13]. This may have occurred because hospice is obviously a team effort and ancillary medical personnel are often more involved or more important at times than the primary physician. This secondary role is often difficult for the attending physician and he/she often withdraws. It is important to recognize that the doctors' skill, experience and ongoing relationship with the patient facilitates and maximizes the effect of the whole hospice team. Terminal care, wherever it is provided, 'must be integrated with the best of medicine. The role of the physician is not diminished when focus shifts from curing to caring and when the goal is enhancement of the quality of the patients remaining life, rather than its prolongation' [14].

The whole person attempting to maintain physical, social and psychological integrity must be considered by the physician. The doctor will be expected to do this while presenting the diagnosis, assisting the patient to live with the cancer, being there during the final stages and at the same time being available to the family. Stephen Hersh describes in great detail the role of the physician in cancer care and his chapter is strongly recommended reading for any doctor practicing in this area [15].

As we have briefly discussed, families are effected by and will respond to the stress of a serious illness in a member. Timely interventions during the crisis can ward off emotionally painful complications [16]. There are some steps that the physician can take during this time: (1) include the family in discussions and plans during the course of the illness, watching for inevitable changes of attitude toward the patient and marked changes in the member's moods or behaviors; (2) help other medical personnel understand the family's responses to prevent negative staff reactions and to facilitate staff support of the patient and family; (3) watch for chances for the family to express fears and concerns as this may minimize acting out in the future, and (4) be ready to make a referral for mental health services if a serious change in family dynamics is noted.

Guidelines for physicians

Patients are considered eligible for hospice care when they are no longer under aggressive treatment for cure of their disease which is progressing despite therapy, and when their life expectancy can be measured in weeks or months. The intent is not to prolong life and, even more to the point, the intent is not to prolong dying. The decision to explore hospice care can be made by the patient or family with input from the primary care physician or oncologist. The referral can be made by the primary care physician, family members, friends, clergy or other health professionals. A member of the hospice care team will make an assessment visit to understand the patient's illness, present physical status, symptoms, problems faced by patient and family and available support system(s) [7]. This assessment will help determine the appropriateness of the referral.

Traditional medicine leans toward aggressive treatment to the end. Knowing when to discontinue aggressive treatment for cure and shift to palliation for symptom control is frequently difficult. It should be considered as soon as there is no treatment that will significantly alter the disease. Yet often there is a conflict between giving additional treatment and giving no treatment at all. Patients and families want to do all they can and are afraid that giving up treatment means giving up hope.

All of a physician's schooling and training emphasizes sustaining and prolonging life, thereby making it difficult to accept the concept that, at times, it may be better to do less for a patient. Technology has made it tempting to try aggressive treatments and the uncertainty of diagnosis and prognosis adds to this temptation. Experts who are more knowledgeable in the disease or in the ethical questions surrounding appropriate medical intervention should be consulted. The patient should also be included in the decision and many people are arranging for 'living wills' even before they have a diagnosis that might end in a prolonged death. The physician must find a way to come to terms with these new thoughts and practices. Since no one can meet every need of another, the doctor finding him/herself in situations such as these should be willing to accept consultation and support.

Most patients worst fears center around pain (how much and how will it be endured), discomfort and dependency – not death. They can prepare for the worst and still expect the best if they are kept alert, pain and symptom free and are allowed as much control over their lives and routines as possible [17]. Their desire to recover may be present even with their acceptance of impending death.

Patients in a hospice program are not denied medical treatment. In fact, since the comfort of the patient and family is one of the primary goals, active treatment is provided to control pain and symptoms. This might include antibiotics to treat infections, radiation therapy to reduce pressure caused by growing tumors or implementation of procedures whereby the patient may receive nutritional supplements. A relaxed, pain-free patient is a source of reassurance to the family whereas a suffering patient causes great anxiety and is seen as more of a burden. Removal of physical distress makes the approach to mental, social and spiritual pain easier. The goal is to find the appropriate treatment, one that removes physical distress while allowing maximum awareness.

Wanzer et al. [18], discuss four levels of care that should be considered and discussed with the patient, family and other health care personnel. The general levels are defined as follows: (1) emergency resuscitations; (2) intensive care and advanced life support; (3) general medical care, including antibiotics, drugs, surgery, cancer chemotherapy, and artificial hydration and nutrition; and (4) general nursing care and efforts to make the patient comfortable, including pain relief and hydration and nutrition as dictated by the patient's thirst and hunger. The program must be individualized since every patient is unique to some degree. In some cases the knowledge of the patient's wishes prior to his/her possible incompetency will influence the level of care.

Physicians caring for dying patients might want to accomplish two objectives. The first is to familizarize themselves with existing programs in their community. (NHO publishes a guide to the nations hospices and also has a national geographic directory. They can be reached by calling 703-243-5900 or writing to 1901 North Fort Meyer Road, Arlington, VA 22209.) Doctors should become familiar with the admitting policies, sponsors, philosophy, specific services, fee schedules and expectations of physician involvement. When and if the time comes for a referral, the physician will be well informed and can effect a smooth transition for patient and family. The second is to review and understand their own feelings, beliefs and values surrounding death and dying. They should be able to comfortably answer questions about continuation of treatment, administration of pain medication, decision making, and discontinuation of life support systems. There are no right or wrong answers. Each one of us must be clear about our own standards before the need arises.

These issues are truly medically complicated and emotionally charged. However, when an informed patient and an empathic physician work together, the experience will tend to be the least troublesome and most rewarding.

Importance of communication

Kübler-Ross, a psychiatrist who has intensively worked with and studied the terminally-ill patient, found that most patients knew they were dying, wanted doctors to tell them the truth and were interested and willing to talk about their dying [19]. This was confirmed by others [20–22]. Hackett [23] found that 80% of the dying patients knew their diagnosis and prognosis even though they were not directly told. They were able to pick up subtle changes in behavior in their doctors and family members. Patients, family and health professionals frequently found themselves in conflict as patients insisted their families (who already knew) not be told, family members insisted that the patient (who already knew) not be told and the professional was caught in the middle. Mutual avoidance and this conspiracy of silence tend to cause a breakdown in communication at a time when satisfying communication is particularly important.

One study of patterns of communication revealed that many close family members did not perceive that they had a communicative link to the medical staff at the large, urban university teaching hospital studied [24]. In such facilities, when the emphasis tends to be on the individual and his/her symptoms, rather than on the complex social interaction in a family, misinformation is often spread. It is important for the medical team members to realize that there may be a considerable difference in what they believe they are communicating versus what the patient or significant other perceives.

It was also observed in this study that families often experienced a lack of confidence that they could receive any help from the medical system. This frequently resulted in feelings of hopelessness and helplessness, further removing them from involvement in patient care. Giving family members a role in the care helps relieve their anxiety and lessens feelings of regret and guilt.

Discrepancies were noted in the areas of the patient's knowledge of his/her disease and its implications, and the family's knowledge in the same areas. When open and shared communication was absent, there was excessive reliance on the hospital for patient care and little desire to have the patient at home. This increased not only the medical team's workload and the patient/family isolation but also the cost of the illness.

The doctor can help by telling the truth. The manner of giving information is central. It should be given in person, allowing time for the patient to express feelings and to ask questions. Time may need to be allotted over several days and may necessitate more than one visit before the information can be absorbed. The patient should be prepared gradually if possible, outlining the treatment and offering reassurance that he/she will not be abandoned [17]. Patients are generally more comfortable with their fates when the physician has been honest, yet reassuring.

Health care professionals taking time to communicate and establish relationships with significant others can lay the groundwork for a supportive environment as the patient's illness progresses. When death seems imminent, the family can be summoned and given the opportunity to spend time alone with the patient. Questions should be answered so that they can fully understand and be better prepared to accept the ensuing events. If time is at a premium and if the physician has a lack of training in this area, he/she is advised to refer to a specially trained counselor or therapist.

Hospice effectiveness

Does hospice do what it sets out to do? The data do not give a clear answer. The proponents of hospice care are firm in their beliefs about its effectiveness. They can cite case after case of patients who lived and ultimately died pain-free and happy, of families united after years of dissension and of meaningful last moments together. These cases are anecdotal and descriptive but should not be overlooked as sources of data in support of hospice care. They describe the commitment and dedication of the movement and show unbridled enthusiasm for its continuance.

The hospice movement has attracted the attention of health services researchers trying to understand the merits of hospice care. They are seeking more rigorous evaluation studies in order to determine the proper place of hospice-type services in the health care delivery system.

Of the studies that have been completed, only a few evaluated hospice care in a rigorous scientific way. Two are mentioned here. The UCLA West Los Angeles Veterans Administration Medical Center Hospice Evaluation Study completed in 1984, randomly assigned hospice eligible patients to receive either hospice or conventional care at this center [25]. This center has an inpatient hospice ward established in 1978 for the express purpose of being evaluated. Hospice eligibility criteria were determined by the hospice program at the beginning of this study. Their program provided hospice care in three settings: (1) in a special inpatient unit, (2) at home, and (3) through a consultation liaison team to other inpatient wards.

One hundred and thirty seven hospice patients and 110 control patients and their primary significant other (SO), if any, were followed until the patient's death. The SO for each patient was additionally followed for 18 months during bereavement. Findings showed no association of hospice care with reduced use of hospital inpatient days, therapeutic procedures or cost. However, hospice patients expressed more satisfaction with interpersonal care and involvement in care decisions and their SOs expressed somewhat more satisfaction and less anxiety than did those of the controls. The differences were attributable in part to hospice staff's better meeting the SOs identified needs [8]. Some of these needs were: to be with the patient, to feel helpful, to be assured of the patients comfort and to be kept informed.

The National Hospice Study [26] looked at 40 hospices (20 home care and 20 hospital based) across the country to study the impact of hospice care on costs incurred and on quality of life experienced by terminally ill patients. They found cost savings associated with home care hospices while hospital based hospices were as expensive as conventional care.

Two surveys done at UCLA showed an interest in the inclusion of hospice care in the services rendered by this major university hospital medical center. One survey [27] anonymously surveyed 395 faculty physicians, Department of Medicine house staff, hospital nurses and clinical social workers to determine the need for a hospice program. Of the 243 respondents, 90 % indicated that the hospital needed a hospice program. They felt it should consist of four important components: (1) medical consultation for symptom control, (2) home nursing, (3) other home support services and (4) psychological counseling. There was some disagreement about the form the program should take but most agreed that 'it is a logical extension of quality acute care and an important aspect of medical education'.

The second survey [28] polled 115 patients being treated for cancer at this same medical center. There were measurable differences in their preferences for certain of the ten services they could choose from. However, they reported a high degree of likelihood of using the services if they were available. The following five services ranked as the ones patients were most interested in: medical control of symptoms; home nursing care; nutritional evluation; occupational, physical and speech therapy and psychological counseling.

In a personal communication, Ira J. Bates, Ph.D., M.P.H. of the National Hospice Organization, stated that NHO believes it is important to emphasize that hospice sees the unit of care as the family and gears its interventions to that end. NHO also conducts a variety of training events all year around the country for continuing education credits for physicians, nurses and other providers. They believe they have taught non-hospice personnel the art of pain and symptom control. Perhaps this accounted for the results of at least one study that showed no differences between types of care in the population evaluated [29].

To summarize, hospice strength seems to lie in the following areas:
1. identification of the unit of care as the family;
2. offering psychosocial support usually not available as part of conventional care, particularly to family members;
3. offering patients more involvement in decision making;
4. specially trained staff and volunteers; and
5. offering education and consultation to non-hospice health care providers.

There are certain patients who are most likely to benefit from this specialized care. Patients who live alone or whose primary caregiver is employed will be more likely to elect care in an inpatient unit. Those with adequate supportive care often choose home care programs. Some families will seek assistance from an inpatient hospice when the caretaking burden becomes too great at home. The severity of functional and nursing care problems at the time of the hospice admission helps determine the type of program chosen. Additional findings from the National Hospice Study [30] showed that women are more likely to be cared for in the home when they were patients and there appears to be a definite relationship between family support and the level of care needs that is frequently altered by the decision to end aggressive treatment.

Hospice must be seen by providers of health care as a viable option for these persons depending upon their individual beliefs, lifestyles and value systems. Any program needs to reflect the uniqueness of the community and its involved individuals. It would seem to follow then that if patients and caregivers can be in an environment that identifies and meets their needs during the end stages of life, they will be more satisfied, less anxious and easier to manage in our existing health care system.

Regulation and reimbursement

The rapid growth of hospice suggests that it has struck a responsive chord in regard to the care of the terminally ill. Like any program or organization on an upward climb, this movement needed to establish regulations and reimbursement policies.

According to the National Hospice Organization 19 states now have some form of licensure and the Joint Commission on the Accreditation of Hospitals (JCAH) has established hospice accreditation standards. These standards were developed between 1981–1983 under a Kellogg Grant. They were compiled from a consensus of standards submitted by organizations in the health care field and are now the only standards used for all types of hospice programs. All hospice programs are surveyed by JCAH before accredition with only one prerequisite. They must be licensed if their program is in a state requiring licensure.*

1982 saw an amendment to the Social Security Act that provides federal reimbursement for hospices under Medicare. It is part of the Tax Equity and Fiscal Responsibility Act (P.L. 97-248, Section 122). This will be a 3-year experiment, through October 1986, with requirements for a quality assessment including evaluation of cost which will help determine whether to continue further hospice benefits [31]. Both the UCLA [25] and the Brown [26] hospice evaluation studies looked at cost effectiveness. Neither found hospice more cost effective when compared to conventional care for the terminally ill.

The majority of hospices in the U.S. provide care through traditional reimbursement methods. These include donations and increasingly common payments by third party payors such as health insurance plans. The majority of the more than 1300 hospice programs are not certified providers, which prevents them from receiving Medicare reimbursement.

---

* For further information call or write to Barbara McCann, JCAH, Hospices, 875 North Michigan, Chicago, IL 60611, 312-642-6061.

Keeping these considerations in mind it is clear that the consumer needs to exercise caution in choosing a hospice program. It is advisable to look closely at such things as physician involvement and other stated benefits.

Concluding comments

In light of the previously discussed research findings it seems that hospice programs unquestionably fulfill needs of terminally ill patients and their family members when these needs are identified. The most effective model for the delivery of hospice care would appear to be one that combines resources of an existing hospital with those of an existing home health agency. This would give access to ancillary services when needed and would provide a multidisciplinary team in either location.

The emphasis of hospice care is on family involvement and a team approach to provide patients with continuity of care, thus avoiding feelings of abandonment. This approach helps to find a much needed balance between dignity, privacy and freedom of choice. It can also offer opportunities for the patient to participate in research projects, if available, that aid in the fight against cancer [32].

Some problem areas still to be reconciled include: finding ways to maintain a link between the oncologist and the hospice M.D.; decision-making in regard to cessation of aggressive treatment; establishment of consistent guidelines for determining eligibility for hospice care; and findings ways to improve cost effectiveness.

Most hospices offer bereavement services, benefits of which still remain to be evaluated. The UCLA Study additionally found that fewer than one fourth of the surviving caregivers participated in bereavement activities that were offered [33]. One reason was to avoid the painful feelings they experienced by returning to the place of the death. Perhaps a hospice that is part of an acute-care hospital would experience better attendance at bereavement functions if they were held elsewhere.

The physician considering referral of a patient to a hospice must above all know the answer to the question: Will *this* hospice contribute to the 'quality of life' of *this* patient?

Acknowledgement

I am grateful to the following colleagues for their editorial assistance: Patricia Ganz, M.D.; Marge Lewi, M.A.; and Jeffrey Wales, Ph.D.

References

1. Ariès P. 1982. The Hour of Our Death. Random House, New York.
2. Fischer W. 1980. Hospice care of the dying and their families. In: Pain, Discomfort and Humanitarian Care. Lorenz K, Bonica J (eds). Elsvier, North Holland, New York pp 329–338.
3. Maddison D, Raphael B. 1972. The family of the dying Patient. In: Psychosocial Aspects of Terminal Care Schoenberg B et al. (eds). Columbia U Press, New York, pp 185–200.
4. Saunders C. 1977. Dying they live: St. Christophers Hospice. In: New Meanings of Death Feifel H (ed). McGraw-Hill Book Co, New York, pp 154–179.
5. Parkes CM. 1974. Comment: Communication and cancer – a social psychiatrists' view. Soc Sci Med 8(4):189–190.
6. Cassileth B, Donovan J. 1983. Hospice: History and implications of the new legislation. J Psychosoc Oncol. 1(1):59–69.
7. National Hospice Organization. 1982. The basics of hospice. NHO, Arlington, VA.
8. Kane R, Klein S, Bernstein L, Rothenberg R, Wales J. 1985. Hospice role in alleviating the emotional stress of terminal patients and their families. Med Care 23(3):189–197.
9. Fulton R, Gottesman D. 1980. Anticipatory grief: a psychosocial concept reconsidered. Br. J Psych 137:45–54.
10. Lack S, Buckingham R. 1978. First American Hospice. New Haven, Conn.: Hospice. Inc.
11. Ganz P. 1983. Models of hospice care. Unpublished.
12. Sontag S. 1978. Illness as Metaphor. Farrar, Strauss and Giroux, New York.
13. Torrens P. 1985. Hospice programs. In: Cancer Treatment. Haskell C (ed). W.B. Saunders Co., Phila., PA, pp 963–971.
14. Saunders C. 1981. The Hospice: Its meaning to patients and their physicians. Hospital Practice pp 93–108.
15. Hersh S. 1982. Psychosocial aspects of patients with cancer. In: Cancer Principles and Practice of Oncology. DeVita V et al. (ed). J.B. Lippincott Co., Phila., PA, pp 264–277.
16. Olsen E. 1970. The impact of serious illness on the family system. Postgrad. Med 169–174.
17. Carey R. 1975. Living until death: a program of service and research for the terminally ill. In: Death: The Final Stage of Growth. Kubler-Ross E (ed). Prentice-Hall, Inc. Englewood Cliffs, NJ, pp 75–86.
18. Wanzer S, Adelstein S, Cranford R, Federman O, Hook E et al. 1984. The physician's responsibility toward hopelessly ill patients. N Engl. J Med 310(15):955–959.
19. Kubler-Ross E. 1979. Death and Dying. MacMillan Co., New York.
20. Feifel H. 1965. The Meaning of Death. McGraw Hill Book Co., New York.
21. Krant M. 1974. Dying and Dignity: The Meaning and Control of a Personal Death. Charles C. Thomas, Springfield, Il.
22. Hinton J. 1979. Comparison of places and policies for terminal care. Lancet pp 29–32.
23. Hackett T. 1976. Psychological assistance for the dying patient and his family. Ann Rev Med 371–378.
24. Krant M, Johnston L. 1978. Family Members perceptions of communications in late stage cancer. Int J Psych. Med 8(2):203–216.
25. Kane R, Wales J, Bernstein L, Leibowitz A, Kaplan S. 1984. A randomized controlled trial of hospice care. Lancet 1:890–894.
26. Greer D, Mor V, Birnbaum H et al. 1984. Final report of Natl Hospice Study. Brown University, Providence, R.I.
27. Ganz P, Breslow D, Crane L, Rainey L. 1985. Professional attitudes toward hospice care. Hospice J 1(4):1–15.
28. Rainey L, Crane L, Breslow D, Ganz P. 1984. Cancer patients attitudes towards hospice services. Cancer 34(4):181–201.

188

29. Kane R, Bernstein L, Wales J, Rothenberg R. 1985. Hospice effectiveness in controlling pain. JAMA 253(18):2683–2686.
30. Mor V, Wachtel T, Kidder D. 1985. Patient predictors of hospice choice, hospital vs. home care programs. Med Care 23(9):1115–1119.
31. Osterweis M, Solomon F, Green M (eds). 1984. Bereavement: Reactions Consequences and Care. Natl Academy Press, Wash., DC.
32. MacDonald N. 1984. The hospice movement: An oncologists view point. Cancer 34(4):178–182.
33. Kane R, Klein S, Bernstein L, Rothenberg R. 1986. The role of hospice in reducing the impact of bereavement. Accepted for publication in J Chronic Dis.

12. Cancer Rehabilitation

EDMOND E. CHARRETTE and DAVID M. O'TOOLE

Introduction

Over the years, the word cancer has conjured images of death, pain, suffering and hopelessness. Because of this, the words 'cancer' and 'rehabilitation' rarely are used together. Dr. Charles Moore said, 'While there are several chronic diseases more destructive to life than cancer, none is more feared'. Dr. William Boyd, a noted pathologist, wrote, 'When we think of cancer in general terms, we are apt to consider it a process characterized by steady, remorseless and inexhorable progress in which the disease is all conquering...'.

The key to treatment of cancer involves early diagnosis, aggressive surgical ablation, possibly intensive chemotherapy and/or radiotherapy, and often all in combination. But if a 'cure' is not achieved, the clinician may be guilty of a defeatist attitude. Very frequently we fall into a trap and commit a serious error in clinical judgement. In his classic *Annual Discourse to the Massachusetts Medical Society* in 1976, the distinguished clinician, J. Englebert Dunphy, made the following statement, "The old adage 'He will be dead in six months', or 'I will give him a year to live' is an unforgivable statement for a physician to make. It is unforgivable because there are no valid grounds to make so rigid a prognosis. It may be three months, six months, six years or longer, and one can never be sure" [1]. This uncertainty about the future introduces a ray of hope, however small, for both patient and family. In contrast, whenever a patient has received such a 'death sentence', the possibility of rehabilitation usually is not even considered.

The word 'rehabilitation' means restoring. In a clinical setting, it refers to bringing about improvement of an individual's ability to return to a prior level of social, physical, emotional and economic functioning after some type of injury or illness. Perhaps the best definition is, 'a team approach to assisting the patient/family as a unit of care, to maintain maximal functioning physically, emotionally, socially and spiritually throughout all phases of

Higby, DJ (ed), Issues in Supportive Care of Cancer Patients. ISBN 0-89838-816-3.
© *1986, Martinus Nijhoff Publishers, Boston. Printed in the Netherlands.*

illness'. This goal is best achieved with an approach that is patient/family centered. It is a continuous process that requires periodic evaluation and it must be goal-directed and be modified, as necessary, through periodic evaluation.

Historically, medical rehabilitation is a relatively recent area of serious study when compared to most other fields of medicine. It was through the efforts of Dr. Howard Rusk, during and after WW II, that the concept of rehabilitation was developed in the United States. Unfortunately, during their medical training, physicians have not always been uniformly exposed to solid teaching in the basics of rehabilitation. A shortage of physiatrists in the academic setting, as well as in many communities, has been a contributing factor. The subspecialty of cancer rehabilitation is a much younger field and it would be worthwhile to scan its development through a brief historical review.

In 1964, Freed and Charrette published a paper to justify rehabilitation of patients who had amputation of the lower extremity for malignancies [2]. In 1967, the first program was funded by the United States Vocational Rehabilitation Administration and the Institute for Rehabilitation Medicine, at Memorial/Sloan Kettering Cancer Center under the guidance of Dr. Herbert Dietz. In 1972, the National Conquest of Cancer Program included references to cancer rehabilitation. In 1973, the National Cancer Institute sollicited proposals for demonstration projects in cancer rehabilitation. As recently as 1981 Dietz published *Rehabilitation Oncology,* the first book devoted entirely to this subject [3]. In 1982, Richard Harvey published a paper summarizing 36 program approaches in the areas of cancer rehabilitation [4]. Since that time, there has been increasing awareness of this medical discipline. Despite this progress, it is not unusual for physicians to be unaware that there are special programs for the rehabilitation of patients with cancer.

Traditionally, medical education has emphasized the acute care setting, with the vast majority of time being spent on the acute medical and surgical treatment needs of patients. Comprehensive inpatient rehabilitation medicine has occurred for the most part in separate rehabilitation centers or hospitals, which are seldom closely integrated into the continuum of care of the acute patient. From an educational standpoint also, there has been a misplaced emphasis of rehabilitation medicine as a specialty which deals with neuromuscular, cerebrovascular and orthopedic problems. Finally, until just recently the attitude towards cancer was often so defeatist that most people could not see any rationale for applying the benefits of rehabilitation to a group of patients who if not cured were expected to die in a short time. Presently, cancer patients are achieving more complete and longer remissions and higher rates of cure. Unfortunately, even the patients who are totally cured of their disease are often left with significant functional problems that are simply not addressed after their acute and dramatic problems have been successfully treated.

A brief anecdote illustrates this point very well. A colleague related that he had never considered the need for cancer rehabilitation until he recently had a patient with acute leukemia who was brought into complete remission using an aggressive chemotherapy protocol during a lengthy hospital stay. When he wrote the order to have the patient discharged, he was reminded by the nurse that the patient was now too weak to walk. The physician promptly responded, 'Well, then send him home by ambulance!'.

The attitudes toward the utilization of cancer rehabilitation seem to be evolving very rapidly. The increasing sophistication of patients and their families is exerting pressure on otherwise capable physicians to become aware of the benefits of rehabilitation in general, and cancer rehabilitation in particular. Present trends towards a more holistic approach to medical care, plus the increasing competition among physicians, will result in a more complete model of care with less emphasis on the acute care aspect of medicine. Stricter utilization review in acute hospitals due to the increasing need for cost containment, as mandated by the federal government, will also play a role in moving patients into the rehabilitation setting. It is becoming increasingly apparent that the best 'value for the medical dollar' can be achieved in the rehabilitation area. This is especially true when compared to the dramatic organ transplants and other ultra high technology medical procedures that are reported almost daily in the press. The number of people who have been cured of cancer, or who have long chronic clinical courses with cancers, marked by sequential remissions, is rapidly growing. Many chronic cancer patients live more comfortably and more often with a higher quality of life than many other patients with 'good' chronic conditions such as those involving the heart, lungs, kidneys and nervous system. The proper selection of which cancer patients should have rehabilitation is not easily answered. Before addressing this issue, it would be worthwhile to review the rehabilitation process and the very important areas of functional assessment and problem identification.

Functional assessment, the key to oncology rehabilitation

Rehabilitation promises no cure; in essence, rehabilitation is a 'functional resuscitation'. The main interest of the rehabilitation specialist is in the area of how disease affects function. Hence, the cornerstone of a cancer rehabilitation program is a functional problem identification when the patient is still in the acute hospital. This must be done by a well-trained professional. In this way, the patient is introduced into the system and is directed into the appropriate level of rehabilitation at an early stage. Ongoing functional assessments are performed at appropriate times, so that during the course of the patient's disease functional needs will be identified and the basic problems can be addressed. The assessment tool must identify functional problems, and measure improvement over time. It can also be used as a tool for program evaluation. Lehman and Delisa [5] pointed out in their evaluation of over 800 hospital charts of patients with cancer, that the major problem was the lack of rehabilitation consultation, which resulted in failure to identify functional problems; they advised an ongoing process of staff education to address this deficiency.

A modification of the Long Range Evaluation System (LRES) is the basic functional assessment tool in use on the Cancer Rehabilitation Unit at the New England Rehabilitation Hospital. The LRES was developed and thoroughly tested by Dr. Carl V. Granger and his associates [6]. It is a global tool which makes use of the Barhtel Index, PULSES Profile and the ESCROW Scale. Also, it can be incorporated easily into a computer data system. The LRES chiefly measures tasks and activities which an individual performs within the context of the physical and attitudinal circumstances of his/her own daily life. Disability represents restrictions in the performance of these activities. The three components of the system allow the measurement of a wide range of functional impairments and handicaps.

The Barthel Index measures independence in self-care, bowel and bladder control, and mobility. The adapted PULSES Profile is a more global measure of independence in daily personal care requirements. The ESCROW Scale measures factors that contribute to household and community supports.

The LRES is structured so that it measures change over time. Through the use of periodic assessments, the rehabilitation program can be adapted to the patient's needs in either a stable or progressive clinical situation. The inter-rater reliability is good, and the instrument has been well established and tested for many years.

The use of the Dietz Classification [3], which we have modified to our Oncology Functional Assessment, makes realistic goalsetting possible.

With the Dietz Classification, one has an ongoing monitor of function that is the essence of the system and makes it particularly adaptable to cancer rehabilitation.

Through the use of the Dietz classification, the appropriate rehabilitation stage of the disease can be delineated. There are four such levels of care.

1. *Preventive.* This is extremely important inasmuch as the majority of patients with cancer will fall into this category. They will require some treatment before the development of a potential disability. The appropriate interventions at this stage can prevent contractures, decubiti, deconditioning, immobilization syndrome and frozen shoulders following mastectomy.

2. *Restorative.* At this stage the patient can be expected to return to his premorbid status without any significant handicap. Once again, it is extremely important to assess these patients as early as possible in order to prevent complications and provide necessary supports so that the goal of return to home, work, or school, is realistic.

3. *Supportive.* This stage indicates that the disease has been controlled and that the patient may remain active with known residual disease and possibly a slowly progressive disability. At this stage, the patient can be expected to return to premorbid status for an appreciable length of time. The patients who fall into this category require the most rehabilitation. Also, this is the group which is sometimes overlooked and this results in a great disservice to them. Reasonable and realistic goals may not be fully achieved because of the lack of recognition of problems on the part of the primary care deliverers. As a result, the patient is not allowed the opportunity of being evaluated by a rehabilitation professional.

4. *Palliative.* This is the category of patients who are suffering from increasing disability because of rapid disease progression. There are some basic preventive rehabilitation strategies that could be provided to these people but they are in a hospice-like situation; therefore, an active rehabilitation program is not appropriate.

Following evaluation, the data may be presented to the continuing care coordinator at the acute hospital who then may forward it to a rehabilitation hospital pre-admission team, the Visiting Nurse Association or other caretakers.

Based on the assessment of the clinical situation – the diagnosis, the present status, the effects of treatment and/or complications, the functional assessment and proper oncology classification – realistic goals may be set. This system also allows the clinican to better advise the family and the patient regarding the realistic expectations that should result from the planned therapeutic interventions.

The cornerstone of a good cancer rehabilitation program is 'problem identification' in the acute hospital. This must be done by a trained professional. The patient is then introduced into the system and directed to the appropriate level of rehabilitation at an early stage.

In our experience, the oncology nurse is ideally suited to carry out this functional assessment. They have access to patients as well as to the oncologists and primary physicians. They are also in contact with families so that they have the potential to be educators as well. Finally, they have a working knowledge of prognosis, side effects of treatment, and other technical issues having to do with cancer.

It has been our experience that education is extremely important. Oncology nurses are in an excellent position to educate both families and patients. They can also discuss ongoing problems with all members of the team, as well as the family.

The rehabilitation process – model and components

1. Assessment
2. Planning
3. Implementation
4. Evaluation

The traditional goals of rehabilitation should apply to the patient with cancer. Rehabilitation goals for patients who have functional impairments are to maximize the functional independence for eventual return to home, community, and employment.

There are several significant factors in rehabilitation planning that are somewhat unique to cancer patients. First, the stage of the disease – progressive, cured or stable – is crucial in realistic goal setting. Second, the effect of therapeutic interventions on both the physical and emotional problems of the patient must be considered. These two factors require a flexible rehabilitation system. Third, the highly emotional impact of the disease, on both the patient and the family affects the program. These factors demand a flexible rehabilitation system. Therapeutic measures to alleviate these problems must be part of any effective rehabilitation plan.

Many patients with cancer have minimal rehabilitation needs and only a very basic program needs to be utilized. However, a significant number of patients have multiple functional impairments and require a sophisticated multidisciplinary program. In order for these needs to be met, the patient must enter into a comprehensive rehabilitation program. The essential part of the program is the identification of functional problems. Once the assessment has been completed, problems are identified and the rehabilitation prescription can be formulated. The implementation is then begun and the appropriate services are prescribed. Periodic reassessments then allow the rehabilitation team to closely monitor the clinical course of the patient.

Cancer rehabilitation team

Just as in any other rehabilitation program, the cancer rehabilitation team is multidisciplinary and the role of each member varies with the problems encountered. The basic cancer rehabilitation team consists of an oncologist, a physiatrist, psychiatrist, physical therapist, occupational therapist, speech pathologist, the oncology nurse, chaplain, social worker, and occasionally representatives of other ancillary services such as neuropsychology and vocational counseling. The ideal team should be stable and be considered a specialty team. Not every professional can handle the vicissitudes of dealing with cancer; therefore, it is very important that the team be made up of mature experienced people. Lines of communication between members of the team must remain open at all times.

Whenever there are so many individuals involved in treating a patient, good communication is essential. This is usually accomplished through the team meeting. Usually the physiatrist is the coordinator chairman. The meeting follows a structured agenda. It is at the team meeting that the patient's progress and problems are reported and the program is modified, if necessary. Discharge planning is done by this group if the patient is an inpatient.

Selection of patients

A very important part of cancer rehabilitation concerns the issue of which patients should be selected as candidates for this type of comprehensive therapy. The selection of patients for cancer rehabilitation is both important and complex, but the process should not be a stumbling block that prevents patients from being referred when they have need for such treatment. With modern treatment, there is a wide range of clinical problems that can develop in these patients. Complications of treatment such as infection, nerve damage from surgery, fibrosis as a result of radiotherapy, and the debilitating effects of vigorous chemotherapy easily come to mind. Recent trends in cancer treatment have resulted in intensive combinations of treatment modalities, as well as potent multi-drug chemotherapy protocols. More complications from treatment occur now than in the past when treatment was simpler, but less effective. The general problems of nutrition with difficulty swallowing and resulting weight loss, and the muscle weakness and the other innumerable multi-system effects of long immobilization and multiple surgical interventions, will often make the patient a candidate for rehabilitation. In addition, the wide variety of nervous system complications which are often encountered, such as primary brain tumors that have been debulked, metastatic brain lesions that have responded to therapy, spinal cord compression, cranial nerve and peripheral nerve damage are other types of patients problems that benefit from proper rehabilitative care. The para-neoplastic syndromes can cause a variety of metabolic and endocrinologic disturbances. These syndromes are responsible for a wide variety of problems that are often amenable to rehabilitation efforts after the underlying neoplastic process has been brought under control by effective treatment.

Adequate pain control is essential in order for the rehabilitation process to even begin. All too often, basic cancer pain control measures have not been utilized. Either insufficient doses of pain medication or lack of knowledge in the recent advances in the control of cancer pain result in suboptimal pain relief. Newer methods of pain control utilizing pharmakinetically based dozing are well covered elsewhere in this book. In our program, the preadmission committee evaluates the cancer patient according to the same criteria as the patient without cancer. These criteria include: independent functioning prior to the acute hospitalization, a potentially improvable situation, demonstration of good rehabilitation potential (and at least a reasonable life expectancy).

Since cancer rehabilitation is still a relatively new field with limited literature, there are no hard and fast guidelines in the selection of patients. For example, patients with primary brain tumors are not very promising candidates. If the primary treatment is radiation, the increase in cerebral edema that results from whole brain radiotherapy often is a problem in spite of treatment with high dose dexamethasone. When the tumor has been debulked, however, prior to radiotherapy, the outlook improves. Some of these patients can have a worthwhile remission period that allows them to enjoy life. Likewise, spinal cord compression by neoplasms often result in much better results from rehabilitation than do traumatic spinal cord injuries. In traumatic injuries, the cord is either transected or severely damaged and there is little or no return in nerve conduction below the area of injury. In contrast, certain types of neoplasms, e.g., breast and gonadal cancers, lymphomas, myelomas, etc., can be treated with a combination of one or more of the standard therapies. Decompressive laminectomy is frequently followed by radiotherapy and/or chemotherapy, and in certain situations, a complete remission or even a 'cure' can be achieved. Though these patients often present very much the same as a patient with irreversible spinal cord damage, with proper treatment one can expect some degree of nerve tissue recovery. Thus attention to muscle strengthening and orthoses or other assistive devices may allow the patient to regain the ability to walk. Some patients return to normal ambulation without any need for assistive devices even though they had a clinical presentation that closely resembled serious traumatic cord injuries. Transverse myelitis as a complication of radiotherapy, can give a similar picture. The management of the neurogenic bowel and bladder is best managed by a rehabilitation team. The patient with a pathologic fracture which has been treated with open reduction, stabilization through internal fixation, and often radiotherapy, is a good candidate for careful application of rehabilitation principles, and may gradually return to normal or near normal function. Patients who have had amputations for cancer should not be denied the usual approach of rehabilitation for amputees.

A very important group of patients frequently overlooked as candidates for rehabilitation are those who are suffering from the immobilization syndrome and all of its various manifestations. Typically, in the acute hospital there are those who have been confined to bed and chair in a small geographic area. They are encouraged to remain in this location for the convenience of hospital operations. This inactivity results in rapid muscle atrophy and resulting weakness which is compounded by the debilitating effects of cancer treatment. The philosophy in a comprehensive rehabilitation facility is just the opposite. Patients are encouraged to be out of bed, dressed and are moved around the hospital to therapies and to the dining room whenever feasible.

Psychosocial issues and the hospice concept are discussed elsewhere in this book. Two other aspects of rehabilitation deserve emphasis. They are maxillofacial rehabilitation and ostomy care.

Maxillofacial rehabilitation is an important area not only because of the destructive effects of the cancer, but also the defects and deformities caused by the aggressive treatment modalities that are employed to treat the malignancy. The head/neck area is emotionally charged because is is always exposed. The appearance of this area has significant impact on all social interactions, and is fundamental to communication. These aspects have been well covered in the literature [3, 7, 8]. In addition to the cosmetic problems, impairment of speech, mastication, swalloing, etc., all can result. Thus, rehabilitation through the use of esophageal speech or some of the newer artificial voice technologies are well covered elsewhere [7]. When the hard plate is defective, there is often considerable difficulty swallowing because of regurgitation into the nasal cavity and in addition, speech quality is impaired with nasal sounds; here, an intra-oral obturator prosthesis can be very effective.

The quality of life for patients who have stomas has been considerably improved through the recent advances in specialized training in this area [9]. Entero-stomal therapists apply their expertise to the various problems that can present in patients with abdominal stomas. This allows patients to have a more carefree attitude and more natural life-style. Self-help groups and the ostomy visitor who shares experience and information with the new ostomy patient, serve a very useful purpose. Local ostomy associations have periodic meetings to provide sharing of experience, plus education and emotional support. Addresses of local units can be obtained from the United Ostomy Association, 200 West Beverly Boulevard, Los Angeles, California 90057.

The wise clinician recognizes that cancer rehabilitation is an important part of the spectrum of cancer care. For the proper treatment of this disease, appropriate consultations are needed and patients are then integrated into a cancer rehabilitation program.

198

References

1. Dunphy JE. 1976. On caring for the patient with cancer. Annual discourse. NEJM 295:313–319.
2. Freed M, Charrette EE. 1964. Rehabilitation after Amputation of the lower extremity for malignancy. A. P.M.R.45:564–570.
3. Dietz JH Jr. 1981. Rehabilitation Oncology. Wiley Medical, NY.
4. Harvey RF et al. 1982. Cancer rehabilitation – An analysis of 36 program approaches. JAMA 247:2127–2131.
5. Lehman JF et al. 1978. Cancer rehabilitation: Assesslent of need, development and evaluation of a model of care. A. P.M. R.59:410–419.
6. Granger C, Gresham GE. 1984. Functional Assessment in Rehabiltation Medicine. Williams & Wilkins, Baltimore/London.
7. Gunn A. 1984. Cancer Rehabilitation. Raven Press, NY.
8. McGregory FC. 1951. Some psychosocial problems associated with facial deformities. Am Soc Rev 16:629.
9. Broadwell J. 1982. Principles of Ostomy Care. C.V. Mosby Company, St. Louis.

13. Early rehabilitation in cancer; a case report

ELLEN P. ROMSAAS and H. IAN ROBINS

Introduction

Cancer rehabilitation is a relatively new concept whose development coincides with an improved outlook for patients with many types of cancer. Improved techniques in chemotherapy, surgery, and radiation therapy have contributed to the control and cure of many types of cancer [1]. Early rehabilitation is a basic principle of cancer rehabilitation [2–4], yet most rehabilitation efforts in cancer focus on chronic residual dysfunction following mastectomy, laryngectomy, radical neck dissection, ostomy and amputation [2, 5, 6]. Even these efforts have been limited [8–10]. As effective treatments for advanced disease are developed, an increasing number of patients who will benefit from rehabilitation intervention will emerge. The following case illustrates that rehabilitation can be initiated immediately following diagnosis and can be incorporated into a course of intensive chemotherapy.

Case report

A 28-year-old man with underlying triplegic cerebral palsy developed testicular choriocarcinoma with lung and bulky retroperitoneal node metastases. The patient's disease process was associated with elevated βHCG levels. Shortly after diagnosis, a nephrostomy tube was placed to decompress an obstructed kidney and cytotoxic chemotherapy was begun. At this time he was unable to ambulate with a walker as he had done before this admission and physical therapy was initiated for strengthening and gait training. Chemotherapy was administered during brief, monthly admissions. During this time the patient developed pulmonary emboli. This complication was felt to be in part due to the patient's immobility.

Six months after the initial admission, the patient was hospitalized for 6 months for treatments which included surgery, chemotherapy and intensive

Higby, DJ (ed), Issues in Supportive Care of Cancer Patients. ISBN 0-89838-816-3.
© *1986, Martinus Nijhoff Publishers, Boston. Printed in the Netherlands.*

rehabilitation. Retroperitoneal lymphadenectomy and left nephroureterectomy were performed in order to remove the abdominal mass which had shrunk in response to chemotherapy. Decreased right-sided strength was noted after surgery and was attributed to a right lumbosacral plexopathy secondary to a postoperative retroperitoneal hematoma.

The patient suffered a reactive depression related to this new clinical complication. Treatment compliance was believed to be critical to achieving a cure in this young man. Rehabilitation Medicine was consulted. Electromyography and nerve conduction studies were performed which revealed generalized bilateral peripheral neuropathy. The patient began an intensive restorative therapy program of lower extremity strengthening and ambulation in physical therapy. The patient was able to perform sliding board transfers and to bear weight but the right leg was weak and an ankle-foot orthosis was prescribed for support. Ambulation was not yet possible and a wheelchair was obtained for indefinite use. Occupational therapy initiated at this time focused on activities of daily living and on wheelchair mobility. The patient's mood and attitude significantly improved after the initiation of this program. Ongoing antineoplastic therapy which included chemotherapy, antibiotic support, and medical treatment for severe esophagitis secondary to chemotherapy-induced vomiting was conducted on the rehabilitation unit rather than on the oncology ward. This was to foster the attitudinal motivation felt necessary for the patient to emotionally tolerate the various medical interventions which were necessary.

Three months into this lengthy admission, thoracic surgery was performed to remove masses which had shrunk in response to chemotherapy. The procedure was well tolerated but the patient complained of right leg pain after surgery. Sympathetic nerve blocks and a transcutaneous electrical nerve stimulator were tried without success and pain was then managed with narcotics. Three weeks after this surgery, βHCG levels were found to be normal, indicating that the cancer was no longer in evidence. Ambulation was resumed in a wading tank 3 and 1 half weeks after surgery. Shortly after this period, narcotics were carefully tapered and then discontinued.

After the patient's chest had healed sufficiently, ambulation was resumed on the parallel bars. The wheelchair remained the most useful means of transportation for the patient at that time. A home visit was made by the occupational therapist in preparation for discharge; modifications were made to accommodate the wheelchair and adaptive equipment was recommended for ease in bathing. At the time of discharge after 6 months, the patient was able to ambulate 50 feet with a front-wheeled walker and was independent in his wheelchair on level surfaces. He was independent with assistive devices in activities of daily living. Due to his low level of endurance, he continued physical therapy as an outpatient.

Follow-up for disease continued to show no evidence of recurrence. Progress in ambulation and in lower extremity strength was monitored closely by Rehabilitation Medicine and the exercise program was modified to allow for changes. At the time of this report, the patient has regained premorbid levels of muscle strength in his lower extremities, uses his wheelchair only when tired or for long distances, ambulates 150 yards with a cane, has resumed his part-time work, is independent in self-care and has no evidence of recurrence 24 months after his last surgery. The patient's probability of being cured with such a disease-free interval is in excess of 97% [11].

Discussion

Few reports have been published which illustrate the use of rehabilitation techniques early in the course of cancer therapy. It is vital for medical staff to recognize a patient's disability and rehabilitation potential early in the treatment process in order to initiate prompt referral for rehabilitation care [4]. For our patient, several early indicators were present: the underlying diagnosis of cerebral palsy, the likelihood that mobility status would be compromised by cancer therapy, and the recognition that mobility status had worsened since the onset of disease. Medical staff initiated a physical therapy consult soon after diagnosis in order to improve ambulation skills and to prevent complications secondary to immobility. Occupational therapy was then consulted to assist the patient with independent living skills, a primary area of emphasis for the patient with metastatic disease [12]. Prompt attention to preventing as well as minimizing disability can reduce the degree of disability and also the time needed for recovery [4]. In chronic diseases such as cancer, rehabilitation potential must be evaluated early in the course of the disease so that anticipated deterioration can be prevented or postponed.

In addition to early recognition of rehabilitation potential, the timing of rehabilitation intervention is important. Rehabilitation has begun typically when the medical condition has stabilized. In cancer, however, rehabilitation measures should not be delayed until all specific cancer therapy has been completed [2–4]. Our patient presented with widely disseminated disease which required major surgery and a 2-year course of chemotherapy, eventually achieving a cure. Had rehabilitation intervention been put off until the completion of cancer treatment, more extensive rehabilitation measures would have been required to reach the same goals and a significant amount of time would have been lost. It is contrary to good rehabilitation practice to defer the provision of rehabilitation services until the status of the disease or the question of spread has been determined [4].

The location of rehabilitation services is a third issue. The first orders for rehabilitation intervention can be made during the acute care period before the patient reaches the status of readiness for transfer to a rehabilitation unit [4]. Our patient was hospitalized on oncology, surgery and rehabilitation units in conjunction with his cancer treatment. Physical therapy was initiated on the oncology unit during the patient's first admission which established diagnosis. The rehabilitation program later expanded to include Rehabilitation Medicine, Occupational Therapy and Orthotics. This program was adapted to the patient's cancer treatment and to other hospital units. During the acute phase of his cancer treatment, rehabilitation focused on immediate goals such as lower extremity strengthening, prevention of disuse atrophy, venous thromboembolic disease, and on increased mobility. During the rehabilitation unit admission, the program was intensified and broadened to focus on the return home.

Early rehabilitation may also serve to eliminate the development of periods of hopelessness, despair and frustration which can be associated with chronic disease [4]. Both psychological and physiological benefits can be attributed to the initiation of rehabilitation intervention. It has been recommended that psychosocial support services be routinely available on oncology services [13]. Our patient exhibited depression related to treatment complications. Improvement in mood corresponded to the initiation of an intensive, restorative program. The goals of restoring strength and improving mobility skills provided a very positive focus for our patient during the course of his cancer treatment. The motivation factor was especially important for him since treatment compliance could reasonably be expected to lead to cure and the resumption of his normal activities.

Conclusion

We believe that the early application of rehabilitation principles is a powerful adjunct to the standard medical and nursing care provided to cancer patients. Rehabilitation professionals including occupational therapists can cooperate in the early evaluation of rehabilitation potential, advise regarding the early introduction of rehabilitation measures, and be flexible in providing services to patients in various locations. Early rehabilitation is a powerful adjunct to cancer treatment.

Acknowledgements

The authors wish to thank Marcia Margolis, P.T., Rehabilitation Unit Supervisor, Donald L. Trump, M.D., Associate Professor of Human Oncology and Karen A. Kienker, M.D., Assistant Professor of Rehabilitation Medicine for their review of the manuscript.

This work was supported in part by P-30-CA 14520 awarded by the National Cancer Institute to the Wisconsin Clinical Cancer Center.

References

1. DeVita VT, Hellman S, Rosenberg SA (eds). 1982. Cancer: Principles and Practice of Oncology. Lippincott, Philadelphia.
2. DeLisa JA, Miller RM, Melnick RR, Mikulic MA. 1982. Rehabilitation of the cancer patient. In: Cancer: Principles and Practice of Oncology DeVita VT, Hellman S, Rosenberg SA(eds). Lippincott, Philadelphia, pp 1730–1763.
3. Dietz JH. 1980. Adaptive rehabilitation in cancer: A program to improve quality of survival. Postgrad Med 68:145–153.
4. Rusk HA. 1977. Rehabilitation of patient with cancer-related disability. In: Rehabilitation Medicine, Ed. 4. Mosby, St. Louis, pp 621–642.
5. Burdick D. 1975. Rehabilitation of breast cancer patient. Cancer 36:645–648.
6. Dietz JH. 1981. Rehabilitation Oncology. Wiley, New York.
7. Dudgeon BJ, DeLisa JA, Miller RM. 1980. Head and neck cancer: A rehabilitation approach. Am J Occupat Ther 34:243–251.
8. Burke LD. 1970. Preface. In the Role of Vocational Rehabilitation in the 1980's: Serving those with invisible handicaps such as cancer, cardiac illness, epilepsy. National Rehabilitation Association, Washington, D.C.
9. McAleer CA, Kluge CA. 1978. Why cancer rehabilitation? Rehabil Couns Bull 21:208–215.
10. Perlman LG, Burke LD. 1979. Cancer rehab: New directions and new attitudes. Am Rehabil 4:25–28.
11. Einhorn LH, Donohue, JP. 1979. Combination chemotherapy in disseminated testicular cancer: The Indiana University experience. Sem Oncol 6:87–93.
12. Romsaas EP, Rosa SA. 1985. Occupational therapy intervention for cancer patients with metastatic disease. Am J Occupat Ther 39:79–83.
13. Lehmann JF, DeLisa JA, Warren CG, deLateur BJ, SandBryant PL, Nicholson CG. 1978. Cancer rehabilitation: Assessment of need, development and evaluation of a model of care. Arch Phys Med Rehabil 59:410–419.

Index